A Doctor's Dilemma

A Doctor's Dilemma

Stress and the Role of the Carer

JOHN W. HOLLAND

FREE ASSOCIATION BOOKS / LONDON / NEW YORK

Published in 1995 by
Free Association Books Ltd
Omnibus Business Centre
39–41 North Road, London N7 9DP
and 70 Washington Square South
New York, NY 10012–1091, USA

99 98 97 96 95

7 6 5 4 3 2 1

The right of John W. Holland to be identified as the author of
this work has been asserted by him in accordance with the
Copyright, Designs and Patents Act 1988

A cataloguing-in-publication record for this book is available
from the British Library

ISBN 1 85343 313 6 hardback

Typeset in Minster Book
Designed and produced for Free Association Books by
Chase Production Services, Chipping Norton, OX7 5QR
Printed in the EC by T J Press, Padstow, England

For Ann,

but also to all who take pains to listen and understand.

Contents

Acknowledgements

I wish to acknowledge my thanks to all those who have engaged with me in the journey towards greater awareness but especially to my families: my parents May and Bernard, my sister Hazel, my brother Bernard, my wife Ann and our family.

Of all the others there have been those who have been especially important. I owe a great debt of gratitude to my patients. I have learnt much from them down the years and examples of what they have taught me fill the book, while in the main my mistakes will be known only to them.

A number of people have read my manuscript at various stages and their thoughtful comments have been particularly useful. I especially wish to acknowledge the contribution of my wife, Ann. Besides her long suffering patience with my absorption in writing, she has given me generous help from her own wide professional experience as a Relate counsellor and supervisor, as well as in countless other ways. My sons – John, Peter, Richard and Michael – have added their thoughtful comment and encouragement, and my sister, Hazel Nichols, has given me most generous help with the manuscript.

The doctors who have trained to be family practitioners with me have been a great stimulus, but particular mention must be made of Peter Winfrey and Donald Kruchek who especially gave me encouragement to start writing. My partners, both past and present, Doctors Jim Gillies, Gill Tuck and Amrit Takhar, have each given me so much in many different ways, but not least by willingly letting me have time out on sabbatical from the hurly-burly of family practice.

Psychotherapists Dr Joy Schaverien, John Holden and Sherley Williams, and Doctors Nigel Turnbull, Sunil Weeramanthri, David Evans, Maggie Coffey, Gavin Kelly and Mellany Ambrose have been generous with their comments. There are others who have played a part: Doctors Michael McGregor, Michael Prentice, Malcolm Davies, Kate Wishart, Chris Scarisbrick, Scot Menzies, District Medical Librarian Helen Lycett, my sister-in-law Valerie, Bridget Holland, Clare Wagstaffe, Anne Garrett and, last but not least, Elaine Thurston who undertook the initial typing. They have all assisted in various ways and I wish to acknowledge my gratitude.

Preface

The examples given in this book are taken from real situations, but details have been changed so as to ensure confidentiality. When that has not been entirely possible, material has been used only after receiving express permission from those involved.

Throughout I use the masculine pronoun when referring to the doctor. I am aware that much of a doctor's, counsellor's and care giver's work is high in those skills of nurture and care that are the especial attribute of women and it is only in the interest of clarity, so necessary in the frequent and sometimes complex examples used, that this wording has been followed.

CHAPTER 1

The Background

Do you find that work often overwhelms you and that you seem to have little energy or time for yourself or your family? Is it hard to face yet another night on call? Do you find that angry people seem to make you feel you have let them down? Do highly manipulative people get under your skin and spoil your day? Or perhaps you find it difficult when patients seem to be stuck to their seats and, even when you have given them much more than their allotted time, it seems impossible to get them out of the consulting room door. These can be very real problems.

Perhaps your personal stress level is sometimes so hopelessly high that you feel trapped by your work and even sometimes regret the day you chose your career. Maybe relationships with your partners only serve to increase your stress, and the suggestion that colleagues can be a source of strength and encouragement seems pie in the sky.

Perhaps, too, people with seemingly endless problems daunt you and fill you with feelings of hopelessness and inadequacy. At times you may find yourself feeling trapped, as if stuck in a slough with the mud and mire of your work sucking at your feet, making every step heavier and denying you any real sense of progress.

These are all feelings I have known at one time or another. They can produce a great weariness that seems to sap your strength; but it does not have to be like that. I wish I had known in my early years as a doctor the things I have discovered with time, and which I have now clarified for myself by writing them down.

It has not been an easy task and, in retrospect, there have been three things that spurred me on. First, there was my own stress with work which seemed to be out of proportion, so that work encroached on my private life quite unacceptably. I needed to clarify and refine what I was doing about this. Secondly, there were the reactions of the doctors around me who were training to be family doctors and who began to request that I write a book. Thirdly, once I had started writing, my colleagues who read it were stimulated to make effective changes for themselves. It will clarify the book's purpose to enlarge on each of these in turn.

Initially I believed that work did not have to take so much out of me, and that a better balance between my work and my private

1

life would be more enriching and well worth striving for. In my early days I had sought to reorganize the work itself, but progressively I realized that I must also reorganize myself if my efforts were really to be effective. Here are three situations to give a taste of the sort of experiences that motivated me.

One of my early out of hours' home visits was to a man with what is probably the most unpleasant medical condition of all. He had suddenly developed acute left ventricular heart failure, a condition, as doctors will know, where there is a pooling of blood in the lungs such that fluid collects in the spaces where air needs to be. He was in real danger of drowning in his own body fluids. I sat him up in a comfortable chair, gave him the relevant intravenous injections, and even followed the old physicians' treatment of putting tourniquets on his legs so as to reduce the amount of blood returning to his overloaded heart and lungs. Happily these measures brought him through so that he could be taken to hospital for stabilisation, but it was concentrated work and pressurised by the likelihood that he would die.

Clearly this was a dreadful experience for the man and his wife. She was too shaken even to help by going to the public telephone to call the ambulance. Clearly, too, while in the end I felt a sense of achievement, the circumstances were very different from the hospital facilities I was used to, and many factors added to the stress I felt as the man's doctor: poor light, a room overcrowded with furniture, a too-anxious wife as my only help and a rural ambulance service that took forty-five minutes to arrive.

The second example is also from my early days of working as a family doctor. At that time our sons were still young. Their birthday parties, with their young friends as guests, required two people to run them, and I wanted to be involved. With a one-in-two on-call rota we could not always have the parties in my off-duty time when I was free from emergency on-call work. I remember one Saturday afternoon having to leave in the middle of a party after I had been called by a father for his son who, he said, could hardly breathe. I set off in the car driving safely but quickly. My disappointment at leaving the party was soon overridden as my concern mounted at the thought of what I might find at my destination, and such was the build up of my anxiety, that I all but ran up to the door of the patient's house.

I found the family having their meal. I looked around at their faces searching for the distressed son and, as I could not see anyone wheezing and ill, asked where he was. He was not in a different room struggling for breath, but was there enjoying some toast.

I was to learn that they were on holiday and taking day trips

2

away from home. The son's intermittent, mild asthma had re-curred that morning but they had planned a day at the seaside and did not wish to shorten their day by a visit to the doctor. Now home again, father had made a dramatic overstatement of his son's condition to make sure he was seen as an emergency, because they had planned another long outing the following day. There seemed little respect for the doctor and his family life, only for this man's convenience. I felt misused, demeaned and very annoyed, and these feelings stayed with me for some hours.

My last example is of a recurring situation, so I will take the most recent occasion. Last night I was on call and my sleep was broken by telephone calls and the necessity of getting up to make three night visits. Today I am tired and irritable. My mind is dulled, my humour reduced, and my pleasure in what I do is hard to find. Nevertheless, all today I have been seeing patients for one concern after another. As this is a recurring experience, the ongoing recuperative time left to me is too short. I want to do my job effectively, but to personally take care of 2,000 people with considerable out of hours' work and often working in other people's emotional minefields, means I am physically over-tired and emotionally drained.

These three situations give something of the framework of stress in which doctors work and which result from the various interweaving conflicts in our lives. For me there is the conflict between my wish to be a good and considerate doctor, and my personal need to be considerate to myself. There is my need to care for patients, but also my need to care for my own family. There are the patients' demands on me to do as they wish when they wish it, and which are intensified by their anxiety that they may otherwise die, and my own need to do what I wish to do for my own sake. There is the patients' need for me to do the mun-dane and unpleasant, and my need to be creative in life's dance. There is my wish to be genuine, and the pull of some portions of society to give up and join in manipulation and selfish concern. Conflicts such as these buffet the doctor, but they are themselves both enmeshed and in conflict with the challenges of the doctor's personal growth. The personal nature of his work dilemmas are frequently mirrored in his personal life so that work conflicts are the source of deep and far-reaching stress.

Of course, on top of these pressures is the fact that family practice is changing. For example, politicians are heaping fast imposed new changes on doctoring. The inconsiderate speed of this management strategy is especially stress-producing (Richard-son and Burke, 1991), and patients are similarly having changes

3

imposed on their work by politicians, which mirror those the doctors are experiencing. As a result, the population is becoming resentful, aggressive and manipulative towards anyone in authority with whom they come into contact, and this often means their doctors. And, as if this is not enough, there are the changes that result from technological advances: for example, computers are altering the business side of doctoring immensely. It is as if lists and databases and time management enable the human mind to work at too many things and too quickly for the doctor to maintain a balance. He must face all these intricate matters in his work and also support the population in its attempts to adjust and deal with the stress they feel at such rapid change.

The second motivation to write this book resulted from the responses of young doctors in training for family practice both in England and Canada. These doctors told me that my approach and willingness to consider certain life issues were something that they greatly valued and which they had not come across either in medical books or previous discussions. Their appreciation eventually led to requests that I write them down. This spurred me on.

Certainly the greatest stress of doctoring involves the emotional dimension. A major underlying dilemma is the degree to which a doctor allows himself to become personally involved with the needs of patients, without draining away too much of his own finite inner resources, and without encroaching too much on his sense of well-being. Failure to keep this in balance can easily result in his being over-stressed or, conversely, overly defended. Both these outcomes deny him an ability to relate closely to family and friends so as to receive sustaining nurture in his turn.

Doctors leave their medical schools full to bursting with the detail of physical medicine which they have crammed in during the brief years of their medical course. Partly as a result of this, many leave medical school vowing they will never sit another exam. There must be a whole variety of reasons for this and, of course, a lot of doctors change their minds, but the general feeling is that they have had more than enough of the forced-feeding style and fear of ridicule that surrounds much of medical teaching. As they enter family practice it therefore comes as a severe shock to find that there is a vast field of learning that remains largely untouched and which begs their attention if they are ever to come to grips with human nature. At medical schools, teaching tends – only partly of necessity – to concentrate on the type of understandings about which it is possible to ask questions in the final exams. Also, the student's experience of life is limited by his relative youth and, although some try, there is not enough time to work both on a comprehensive knowledge of physical illness and on a good understanding of human behaviour and the norms of personality development.

And yet a considerable part of a family doctor's work lies in the area of the human psyche. Published estimates are that it is more than 40 per cent (Balint, M., 1957). Patients are not a representative cross-section of the general population. Many attend because psychologically they are stuck in life, and even those with totally physical illness have to adjust to the shock and stress of those physical ills. Slowly, therefore, the family doctor comes to see human psychology as a necessary part of his work – and a rich part at that. This realization usually develops alongside a belief that facing life's conflicts aids their resolution.

However, these realizations take time. Adjusting into medicine is a bit like a marriage. There is a seven-year itch of dissatisfaction until those involved realise they need to dig deeper. Some marriages break up so that digging deeper is avoided for the moment, while others come to grips with it and, as a result, their lives become richer and more exciting.

The third motivation for my writing this book was not so much there in the first place but rather one that spurred me on once I had started. When I had reached the stage of having my thoughts down in draft form, I sought the reactions of my friends and colleagues. I experienced considerable pleasure and reassurance when I found that they had the patience and stamina to navigate through the unpolished and often confused paragraphs, and then went on to give me encouragement. I was struck by the way in which many of them involved themselves in its reading, clearly stimulated to explore further for themselves and to reach for their own greater flexibility and a better balance between work and life in general. For instance, one colleague has said that when first confronted with the draft of this book he felt he did not have time to read it: he was too busy, he had the concentration only for some quick-fix article on a topic that he could rapidly master so as to make a few adjustments here and there, the better to treat his patients. He was far too busy to get into a whole book, even though it was fairly small. He said it was like considering a weekend's holiday in the Lake District: 'It's too far. I've too much to do. Perhaps some other time.'

Then he began reading the book. He said later that it was like being on that holiday in the English Lakes and, when first starting to climb a hill, he would find his muscles complaining and it felt like too much personal effort. 'Why do this to myself? I shouldn't have come. It's not worth it. I don't have time.' But then he found he was dealing with one or two patients differently. They seemed to begin to face up to their problems and take their lives into their own hands. That movement in his work brought him a sense of hope and encouragement. It was as though the view improved as he rose higher up the lower slopes and into the mountains.

Further into the book he began to be concerned. It was involving him more than he had thought. If he restyled his attitude to patients, he then found it affected his attitudes towards his partners, the practice staff and even those at home. This, he felt, was like the challenge of a walk along the top of an arête, with the land falling away steeply on both sides of a mountain crest. But slowly his concerns subsided as the view improved the higher he went, the climb proved safe, and once his muscles were more used to the exercise they stopped aching. Later there was the downhill journey to warmth and sustenance and the promise of the deeper comradeship that follows a day with others in the hills.

It was not that the book gave him another mountain to climb, he said, but rather that it provided a map of the mountains which had mistily confronted him all along. It gave him a sense of knowing where he was and of the routes he could take to progress, a sense of what could be there at the end of the day.

This was his reaction and he wanted the manuscript for others to read so that he could discuss it with them. It was reactions like this that motivated me by confirming the effectiveness of my presentation, and gave me confidence to continue.

Now I am a family doctor and that is the setting for this book. It is a reflective and intimate search into the role of the carer, into the attitudes the doctor may bring to his work, and into society's expectations – all of which affect doctors deeply. However, that by no means makes it applicable only to medical students and doctors. The allied medical professions, such as community and psychiatric nurses, health visitors, midwives, occupational therapists, counsellors, social workers and clergy, all exercise a caring role and will find their conflicts echoed and clarified here.

And there is a reason why family doctoring is a particularly helpful focus for understanding the care-giver's stress. Frequently understandings develop as a result of studying extreme situations. It is as if the exceptional serves to force the main issues out into the open. Family practice is just such an extreme. A doctor's responsibility is unusual in that it extends across the twenty-four hours of each day, as well as covering the physical, social, psychological and clinical areas of caring for adults. Once other professions had continuous responsibilities but now I can only think of one other role in

6

life that is close to this total care, and that is parenting. However, parents care for their own children and do not have the pressure of clinical responsibility. I believe a family doctor's care is unique, and understanding the extreme example of the doctor's role will be of value to other care-givers.

The role of care-giver is stressful, but happily human stress is now becoming a subject that can be talked about. Progressively it is seen as part of everyone's life, a part which, once admitted, can be worked on and adjustments made. And it is just as well, because stress is increasing as more and more is expected from the individual, and society's changes heap one on top of another, each change demanding personal adjustments and producing the stress that accompanies adaptation.

There are different levels at which stress can be understood and therefore differences in the work necessary to ease it. The behaviourist may talk in detail of time management, prioritising, delegation and maintaining good communication (Burnard, 1991). All are certainly important, but these are behaviours that are learnt as if they are externally applied to the individual. However, there comes a time in life when stress is seen to be internal, and that is when people come to look at the well-springs of their tensions (for instance, at the conflicts which prevent people relaxing even when taking well-earned coffee breaks, and when work is both well-managed and shared between adequate numbers of people). It is this level of understanding that this book seeks to explore. Internal stress arises because of the way the individual is, and because of the way he responds to the external pressures of life.

Probably the readers who will relate most closely to this book will be those who have been in a caring role for at least two years; long enough, that is, to have begun to be aware of the internal forces that their work exerts. They will have an approach to life that is willing to question themselves as much as others, and wish to hold themselves responsible for as much of their lives as possible.

In seeking to understand the particular stresses of a doctor in his caring role, it has proved necessary to focus on the doctor as well as the doctored, since work and worker interrelate. It is as if the result is larger than the sum of the two individuals involved. Something goes on between them, such that each builds on the other and creates, as it were, a substance that lies between the two. It is a substance that can tie them together and produce stresses between them that are peculiar to the two. It is this that requires understanding if the carer's stress with his work is really to be eased.

And yet that still leaves the picture too restricted. For instance, what qualities does a young person possess that make him choose doctoring? What are the attitudes in him that lay behind that choice and, now that he is a doctor, make him function as he does? In the carer's past lie clues to attitudes that now lock him into his way of working and which may not be appropriate to the task now at hand. Past experiences have formed his attitudes and bring their own particular stresses.

Patients, too, have backgrounds that shape their expectations. In all, it is as if the patient and doctor are players against a backdrop of expectations, while society, as the audience, makes judgements. The show cannot go on unless both patient and doctor play their part, and the outcome is greater because of the broader interaction with society.

This book is, therefore, about the doctor as a care-giver, his work, the patient, and society. It is not a manual on how to reduce stress and yet it sets in motion adjustments which bring about that result. Deeper understandings both enable a deeper relief of stress and allow greater autonomy, increased effectiveness and a fuller sense of job satisfaction.

To help develop this understanding I give many examples drawn from family medicine. In seeking to understand them I have drawn on insights from other disciplines, notably from the fields of psychotherapy, management and teaching. My experience in practising and teaching family medicine and my work as a diploma member of the Institute of Psychotherapy and Counselling (WPF) have been especially useful. Psychotherapeutic theory and practice lend depth to the understanding of human conflicts.

Doctors, of course, differ both in their understandings and in their style of work. Some doctors choose one route, others another. Some stay more with physical medicine, its facts, tests and X-rays; others vary their focus with management, with committees, or with community work, while others work to develop their understanding of human behaviour. For all, there is a satisfying progression in knowledge and skills. My choice was to develop my understanding of human nature, of man's defences, of what he defends against, and the skills to aid another person's self-discovery.

As this book is an odyssey and a personal way of looking at family practice, it seems to me that some openness about myself would be useful to the reader. After all, it is out of my upbringing and background that these ideas and working methods have evolved and from which my decision to become a doctor arose. Also I wish to illustrate the text with frequent examples. Where these are about interactions between patients and their doctors, the material will inevitably involve the doctor's attitudes and feelings and, therefore, some background to the doctor will increase the understanding of the dilemmas. With this in mind I have appended a brief autobiography.

It is significant that there came a point in my writing when my time-keeping in relation to surgery appointments, while never particularly bad, improved noticeably and my own stress with consultations was reduced. At the same time a larger number of patients than before openly expressed their appreciation of their time with me. I see this as a direct result of defining my role, clarifying what is necessary and useful, and removing the unhelpful and the clutter.

I have given references to other people's work where I am conscious that they have fed me with ideas. There will be other concepts that I have absorbed but am no longer able to say from where they first came. While the Bibliography gives the source when I know it to be other people's work, I would like to add that I tend to value ideas, not only when they first impinge on me and open some door of understanding, but also when those ideas are framed in such a way that they entice me to pass through the door to what lies in the next room. This is often as a result of a particular clarity or imagery. I have therefore also chosen the works listed in the Bibliography because of their presentation of ideas.

I am aware that my way of thinking is different from some people's. A French polisher makes two sorts of movement on the wood surface with his polish pad. One movement is straight up and down the full length of the surface, and the other is in repetitive small circles that steadily work over the whole area, but in that process, passes over any one place several times with different circles of the pad. It seems to me that this latter movement represents my natural way of thinking. It then takes considerable effort to put my thoughts into linear expression. In writing this book I am aware that where I have been reaching beyond what is clear to me (and therefore into what I regard as the more interesting areas), this circular way of thinking has been more apparent, and while some may have no problem with a presentation of that nature, others find it less easy to follow. I have worked to make my presentation acceptable to the majority.

Most people who pick up a book of this kind begin by dipping into a chapter that has particular relevance for them. However, in this book there is a progressive build up of theory and understanding and so, once readers have initially dipped in, I hope they will then read from the beginning.

CHAPTER 2

A Doctor's Dilemma

Whenever young doctors take part in free-roaming group discussions and tutorials, a recurring theme is the distress they experience in their work with patients. This is first voiced by the more open individuals and, significantly, almost universally by those doing a paediatric placement where human distress at the bedside of a dying child and with the parents of dead or dying children is at its most unbearable. The doctor must throw up high defences to deal with the emotion surrounding these events. Frequently, his own emotions dig more deeply into him because he has a sense of responsibility that, as the patient's doctor, he should somehow have saved them or, at the very least, should be able to ease the relatives' distress. Of course, in reality he cannot, but assumptions like these will add the distress of guilt to the other emotional burdens he carries, for he too is party to these events.

Human assumptions start to form with the experiences of childhood, and many of them are carried on into the young person's chosen field of work. There they shape the doctor's attitudes and beliefs, and help form his strong and precious youthful motivations. But at the same time these same young people are in the middle of developing and refining their personalities. They are into a process that includes letting go of childhood attitudes so as to make room for altered perceptions and personally chosen values. There is therefore an enormous amount of high priority, painstaking and personal work taking place in the young doctor just at the time when he begins to face the challenges of his chosen profession. But these two priority areas, which both involve considerable internal change, seem to make demands which can seem impossibly conflicting. An example will help to flesh out the young doctor's situation.

Years ago a young hospital doctor put a great deal of effort into the care of a patient with kidney failure. He had thoroughly informed himself of the detail of the treatment of acute renal failure by peritoneal dialysis which had then only just been pioneered and published, and had himself arranged for the hospital to obtain all the necessary equipment. However, it later became necessary to transfer the patient to another hospital and it surprised everyone, including the doctor himself, how possessive he had become as he tried everything to prevent the patient's transfer. Only later, and

10

after considerable discussion, did it become clear that he had a personal need to take special care of this man because years before, and long before there had been effective treatment, his own father had died of renal failure. His need to care for this patient was a reflection of the time when, as a little boy, he had longed to save his father's life. It had also been this experience which motivated him to become a doctor in the first place.

This is an obvious example of how the understanding of a doctor's motivations can uncover conflicts that centre on the work he has chosen to do. Allen has pointed out the relatively early age at which many doctors decide on their careers, and the frequency with which they say this was to 'fulfil the aims and aspirations of others' (1988). While there will be many strands to the choice of medicine as a career, people frequently choose their work because of deep needs that demand satisfaction, rather than from mature interest. These needs are usually confusingly composite and not easily understood, but what is apparent is that the unravelling of motivations will necessitate a doctor considering his past life experiences – even though they occurred long before he even contemplated the career he would follow.

Another example will shed more light on this. It is taken from J. G. Ballard's book *The Kindness of Women* (1991), the sequel to what is perhaps his best-known book *Empire of the Sun* (1984). It is an autobiographical account of his adjustment to life following his imprisonment in China by the Japanese in the Second World War. He was still a boy, reeling not only from many experiences of violence, death and human destructiveness, but also from feelings of impotence at his inability to relieve the suffering he had witnessed. He had developed a street-urchin-like 'know-how' in the prison camp which stood him in good stead on many occasions but, highly refined as this had become, it did not enable him to do more than observe when he was present at the death of a young Chinese boy by slow torture. It was as if he was tainted by his experiences and left to carry heavy feelings of guilt. Could he only use his *savoir-faire* to save himself, leaving others to die?

He chose to study medicine. The decision seemed to come out of the blue, but he was later to find that anatomy, which involved the dissection of human bodies, so dramatically confronted his raw memories of death and torture in the prison camps that those memories returned to disturb and preoccupy him. He therefore pulled out of that career and turned instead to writing.

Years later he was to write of those wartime childhood experiences (Ballard, 1984). It was as if he had eventually been able to assimilate the suffering and his own feelings of guilt, and to face the emotions and achieve integration of his past with the person he now was. A deep need to face these things had been there in his teens – evidenced by his choice of medicine with its promise of power over other people's pain, and which might have relieved him from his deeply painful childhood sense of impotence and guilt. But it was, nonetheless, a career choice that too soon heaped more suffering – albeit other people's – onto his shoulders. It was like rubbing salt into still raw wounds. He could not yet cope with more distress, and so he retreated from medicine and gave himself a more leisurely developmental journey towards his personal healing.

Although few will have had the dramatic experience of being a Japanese prisoner of war, this example further illustrates the doctors' dilemma. On the one hand many doctors have an impelling necessity to sort out and integrate the feelings and experiences that have unconsciously drawn them into their careers and yet, on the other hand, they are hardly able to face the pace of integration which dealing with so many other people's pain forces on them. When a doctor is young, his feelings are raw. For him to make the journey of sorting his own emotionally charged conflicts at all, he must do so at his own pace, or he will shut off in sterile, debilitating defensiveness. It is probably true that the more personally motivated he is, the more sensitive he will be to other people's situations, and the more essential it is that the speed with which successive patient distresses come his way should be his own. His personal work cannot be undertaken at a pace appropriate only to the needs of his many patients. This is a dilemma at the core of his being.

Even as a student, the doctor-to-be begins to discover conflicts between his own needs and those of patients. Many of these conflicts belong to all young people moving into adulthood, while others are peculiar to doctoring. And yet, just as it was for the two people already quoted in this chapter, it is usual for the conflicts in the area of the doctor's work to mirror those in his personal life. For the doctor, his work is at once so central to life itself and so intrinsic to his own person that it cuts straight to the undefended centre of his being.

There is one dilemma that is common to everyone and it centres on the young person leaving home. University terms minister to a new student's ambivalence about leaving home by the three-times-a-year return to living back with the family. This to and fro softens the process of 'the loosening of apron strings' and doctors have, of course, all been students and experienced this gentler separation, so they may be less aware of its importance to them. Clearly it is a part

12

of the process of growing up. No doubt, as a small child, the doctor was told not to touch the fire, nor was he allowed to cross the busy road on his own. He was protected. However, parental protection will not have prevented his much-loved cat from dying, and in such circumstances he was perhaps gathered up onto grandad's lap to cry. If at first he defensively pretended indifference to the loss of his pet, then on that lap, in the safety and comfort of closeness, he found another who could understand and share his feelings, confirming for him their reality and value. Any tendency to cover up his feelings was nursed away for his inner reality to find its place. He was not rushed, and the process of accepting his distress could be complete.

As they get older, each young person's journey to move out of the family and face life for himself will be different, but it will always include a personal experience of separation. It will include moving out from the protective cloak of family as well as letting go various family beliefs and values so as to free himself to find his own.

Not only will a young person have to question and reconsider his immediate family's ways of thinking about things, along with their assumptions and expectations, but also he will often have to free himself from his grandparent's hopes and expectations, as they will have shaped those of his parents. If, without questioning, his parents merely made the grandparents' attitudes their own, then the young person will be questioning the fixed and powerful *raison d'être* of at least two previous generations. Such circumstances demand that he discover and understand his family's past. For instance, doctors have frequently come into medicine because of a deep need to be in control of the feelings produced by illness: they have an inner need, developed through their upbringing, to control physical suffering and to prevent death with its pain at loss. As a result, although outward control (let alone inward) is largely illusion, nonetheless many will try. In my own family, my grandmother lost all her nine babies before my mother's birth. Her grief at such remorseless loss made her turn inwards and become unavailable to the three later children who survived. This could well have created a half-formed, unspoken wish that there might be a doctor in the house to 'prevent' such an experience happening again; to stop death, to take care of the mother's mental suffering, and to prevent the resulting emotional deprivation to the remaining children. In retrospect it seems to me that such unspoken feelings and assumptions resulted in my mother's pressure on me to be a doctor.

These chains of cause and effect are common in Dr Norman

Paul's experience. He focuses his effective and well-recognised family therapy work on past loss and griefs that have remained unspoken and therefore have not been worked through. Once brought into the open and talked about, these disrupted families move on into more appropriate response and adaptation (1975). Similarly, unconsciously held reasons for becoming a doctor can produce powerful needs to prevent death, and are especially demanding because they are unconscious.

Changes in a young doctor's beliefs and attitudes will often involve assimilating and sorting deep conflicts such as these which are rooted in their families upbringing. At times this will involve rejecting a parent's strongly held belief or wish for his offspring. Parental support is ambivalently both required and rejected. At the young adult stage in life there are kaleidoscopic mixtures of feelings like this which, to a large extent, effectively disarm young people throwing them into disarray.

Through understanding and challenging assumptions and attitudes such as these, the doctor's developmental need will succeed in pushing him out into the world to discover and take hold of the person that he is and to own his own authority. It is naturally a long-drawn-out process. There are some who say they are not free until after their parents are dead. Yet others feel they cannot break free because their parents died before they were able to accomplish this freeing of self. But although this is a life-long process, in a young adult it is an acutely pressing need that demands emotional sensitivity, and it is highly unlikely that the facility of grandad's knee (with time given to focus on the younger person's concerns and feelings) will be available to him. Nor is it likely that new relationships will have developed that are, as yet, as trusted or as facilitating. Nevertheless, for the young medical student who is well into the energy-consuming processes of the personal development necessary for his age, and whose life is devoid of adequate supports or of the strength derived from experience, there flows a succession of other people's distressing feelings and the raw emotions of his chosen career. These seem to pack themselves into his day, one on top of another, too fast to contemplate, and so many, so fast, demand that he distance himself behind the white coat of one who seems to understand illness, and who may be presumed to prevent death. He is pressured to join a club of people whose membership enables him to enter the hospital wards not as a patient – a person who can be ill, disabled or in pain – but quite, quite separate, as 'doctor'. He puts on a cloak of defence against human emotions, which too-frequently also separates him from his own tender growth and sensitivity.

The disturbing emotions that arise out of a doctor's work will frequently involve personally sensitive areas of his being. For instance, he must face the sharp realisation that life is of limited span. This is normally faced at around mid-life; younger people keep it at a defensive distance. I first became aware of this in my early days at medical school when I entered the dissecting room. I felt disquiet but did not know why. I found myself somehow needing to prepare myself to go through the swing doors to the room, yet did not know what to prepare myself for, let alone how. Three of us arranged to go into the room together. In retrospect it was as if each needed the others for support. There were rows of tables, and each had a cloth spread over what was unmistakably a body. Some looked different, and it dawned on my numbed mind that these bodies had already been partially dismembered. At some tables there were students at work: some were grouped around the head and others around a leg or the chest. My eyes were drawn to these tables. Here there was activity and a focus on anatomy that enabled me to move away from feelings into thinking; away from the shapes I knew as human and sensitive, and into thoughts about what went on in the body, to a division or small part of the whole, into anatomy. There were bits of tissue that had been dissected and put to one side. I did not want to see that. I focused on a dissected area of nerves and blood vessels which I could mentally busy myself with, rationalising, and so escaping from my feelings.

We did not stay long, and coming out of the room I experienced a sense of relief mixed with elation. In retrospect, I see I had quickly found the defences I needed at the time to blunt close confrontation with death and the human body's inevitable decay. Nevertheless, for me that dissecting room, situated as it was out of the way on the top floor, always seemed like a brooding presence that hung over the building, so that it was a conscious relief when my studies changed and I began to attend the hospital itself and deal with people who were alive.

Yet as the doctor's medical training unfolds, he again begins to meet situations that are well ahead of his own life experience and out of time with his personal maturity, and where life does not turn out as people wish or expect. Deformities and illness become the focus of his study. These range from those that are just inconvenient to those that leave the patients dead or their lives badly disrupted. And there is also dramatic emotional pain that floods the doctor's own feelings. It cannot be seen, nor is it easy to define. Its depth can only be guessed and fear seems to lurk in its deepest recesses. These experiences creep into the doctor's life just as he leaves home and school and is needing time for himself, time to discover who he is and how he personally feels now that he is away from the guiding hand and steering concern of his family, teachers and childhood friends. Better to think of such feelings as signs of weakness or vulnerability and to consider them as unhealthy, and so feel justified in judging it prudent to put them aside to be ignored. Most young people have not yet personally and fully experienced their depth. They dimly sense they will one day be theirs, but meanwhile they defend themselves by pushing them well away, and considering that 'normal' life consists only of 'healthy' enjoyment.

There are many experiences of this nature which are unavoidable for a doctor in training. They are forced on him by the nature of the job in hand. They bring feelings that belong in other people's lives, but they swamp him while he is still young and lacks the maturity to handle them. He must learn to defend himself against their onslaught.

Human defences are a valuable necessity and are erected against distressing experiences which people find too immediately overwhelming to handle. But the stress of too much, too quickly, may force the response of blanket defences which a more steady introduction would not warrant, and which can result in those defences being maintained for far longer than is either necessary or appropriate. Not only this, but blanket defensiveness also spills out into other areas of life, forcing insensitivity, loss of awareness and loss of appreciation of that which is fine and brings sustenance to the soul. Moreover, building high walls consumes considerable energy – and it takes a similar energy to liberate oneself from them later. It requires time, sensitivity and gentleness even to approach those issues once more. Meanwhile the over-defensive person is less able, so that his effectiveness suffers and his personal development can be delayed. It can therefore be considered a calamity when overload drives someone into inappropriate, excessive and long-held defensiveness. In more reasonable circumstances, human defences can be raised and lowered appropriately, and people are consequently able to respond flexibly or firmly to the changing events of life just as they wish. It is healthier and more comfortable in the longer term to remain open to feelings, sampling them, and more fully integrating one's experience.

Considerable energy can be expended in maintaining an undue defensiveness. For instance, a predecessor of mine in family practice found patients so demanding that he decided to move to Tasmania. There, he reasoned, people would be paying for their doctoring and that would limit their demands. He uprooted himself and his family, and off he went. Later he explained that, far from limiting patient demands, it seemed to make them more persistent: as they paid directly for what they got, he felt it even more difficult to resist their demands. He began to see that the change needed to be in himself, and he returned to practice in England. But what lengths he had gone to in order to avoid making any change to his own difficulty in saying 'No'. The effort he put into moving to another country was tremendous, and it took all this before he was willing to see his problem as internal and, therefore, within his ability to resolve. All that energy became available for other purposes when he let himself change, but his resistance to letting go of his defence had been equally enormous.

On the one hand, a doctor's own development requires that he re-examine his defences and develop an ability for openness and sensitivity to himself and others; on the other, the onslaught of patient needs and distresses that he meets in his work will often necessitate that he defend himself so hugely that those defences will overflow inappropriately into his private life. So it was that in my first years in family practice an old college friend, who had emigrated to Canada, paid us a visit and, in the direct way Canadians have, asked me: 'Are you happy, John?' I remember it so very clearly. I had been absorbed in watching my eldest son's performance at his sports afternoon. Now, suddenly, I was riveted. What a question to ask. I did not want to hear it – and certainly did not want to answer it. I forget just how I answered – something about early days and getting used to my work. The truth had, however, dawned on me in that moment, that work was flooding me: needy people wanting my time; distressed people wanting to off-load their distress; ill people needing my action; manipulative people pushing and pulling; people coming to see me; people pressing for me to go to them; people coming down the telephone wires into my own home – and even my bedroom. People, people, people. I wanted to be of use, but this was madness. Their constant demands, so it seemed to me, took priority and left me little energy or ability to give time or attention to those I loved. Not only were my family and friendships overrun but also my own self, my sense of being. And yet, alongside this, I had been brought up with the attitude that to be busy in the service of others was good and this was unconsciously used as a defence against making changes in my attitudes and behaviour, and my excessive work pattern.

I heard the story of a doctor's small son being asked what he would be when he grew up. 'Oh,' he said with the certainty that springs from experience, 'I'll be a patient, then I can see my daddy.' My situation was certainly not unique. But would I defend my position, and the attitudes that lay behind all this, by comforting myself that I was no different from my colleagues, or would I strive to make changes by first understanding what was involved?

Professor Robert Lane (1993), after reviewing research into the factors relevant to a human sense of well-being, concludes that a satisfying family life is the most important. Frequently doctors need reminding that a far more usual and normal professional life is one in which work finishes on going home at, say, six o'clock, and only starts again on leaving in the morning – and this generally for only five days a week. The family doctor's work is far from reasonable or normal in this day and age. He even expects his work to erode time with family, but with that loss his sense of well-being goes as well.

Professor Lane was of course considering research into society, in general, but there is a sense in which the problem is greater for the helping professions. They are a self-selected group which frequently means they share an inner need to take care of people. How hungrily needy patients hook into a doctor's own need to help and be of use. The two lock together, one helping and the other being helped. The doctor is transfixed by his own need and will often collect more and more needy patients, becoming ever more grossly overloaded. Such a doctor resents his patients but fails to see he is collecting and keeping them to satisfy a deep need in himself.

The condition is self-perpetuating. The more a doctor takes responsibility from people and carries it himself, the greater the burden he carries and the greater the other's impotence, but the greater the patient's impotence and irresponsibility, the more the doctor may feel himself impelled to be responsible for them. In these circumstances it is easy for a doctor to compound the patient's difficulties while producing extra burdens for himself, and both patient and doctor are hampered in their developmental need effectively to shoulder only personally relevant responsibility. The doctor, meanwhile, is more taxingly drawn into his work so that his personal life suffers and he steadily loses his sense of well-being.

The young doctor is often confused by his feelings of responsibility. His own developmental needs demand that he become a responsible adult, but he has not yet defined the boundaries of what being a responsible adult means. He is himself in the process of separating from his parents, of defining himself as an individual and developing close relationships of his own choosing. And yet the succession of distressed people he meets through his work means he must defend himself, or meeting too many perturbing situations and too many people too fast, means he has little time to readjust after work and let his defences down again to his private life's advantage.

This inherent, powerful dilemma for the doctor is one which, in one form or another, remains a central conflict affecting him all his working life. He must constantly make deeply significant adjustments between work and home, day by day throughout his life. Yet work in and around other people's lives so closely mirrors his own personal life that each makes the other more difficult and one seems to flow into the other. He cannot afford to be so overloaded with other people's feelings that he shuts himself off, stressed into becoming defensive and therefore insensitive to himself and his own feelings. He can ill afford to be overwhelmed by the volume of disturbed people pressing in on his developing personality, forcing him to maintain high and fixed defences which shut him off from his private world as well as from the public for whom they are a necessity.

He needs time with his family and chosen friends, to hear their concerns, share their lives and their pain, to draw close in sharing and in involvement, and give and receive life-sustaining, normalising nurture in his turn. He does not need to shut off from his own life's ups and downs because he has been so close to so much of his patients' sufferings that he can bear no more.

He needs to dare to get closer to his chosen partner, and discover with her and with their children the wonder and breadth of mutual togetherness. He does not need, at this time of developing trust and the testing of intimacy, to be loaded with the detail of other people's broken relationships which can scare away his own delicate exploration.

He needs unstressed time to let his new relationships evolve, time free to be himself without the blinkering effects of being too much at other people's beck and call. He needs to be the young person he is, discovering life, rather than pressed into being an all-experienced father-figure, wise beyond his years, to patients often old enough to be his parents or even his grandparents.

He needs time and space for himself, to be able to withdraw a little distance from people who encroach on him, to a position where he can maintain himself. He needs to be able both to be separate and to seek company when, and with whom, he wishes. This sensitive, integrating and personally freeing work must not be swamped by those who give others little space as they manipulate and cajole, as they order and pressurise and attempt to control.

In short the doctor needs the very atmosphere of care and

concern, with time for self and for reflection on his own life, which it is his job to create for his patients. The more sensitively he does his job, the more his own need can be denied. This is a doctor's deep dilemma.

CHAPTER 3

The Nature of a Doctor's Stress

I remember a very stressed man coming to see me. He had come by car along a road he knew well and which had once curled around the countryside following the line of the old hedgerows, but which some years before had been straightened to leave the curves as secluded resting places for motorists. This man's mind had been focused on making good time, and he had assumed one of the resting places meant that he was on a dual carriageway. As a result he had begun to overtake the car in front only to be confronted, literally, by his mistake when he came face to face with a fast oncoming car. He had been very lucky to escape, he said, and if he had not realised already that he must do something about his stress, he considered this experience would have forced him to do so. Stress causes people to shut down their awareness as they try and assimilate the material they are already handling, and in this way – just as it had been for this man – stress can be life-threatening and sometimes, arguably, the direct cause of death.

Stress can certainly be as serious as that, but far more common are the deterioration it causes to relationships at work and at home, a growing inefficiency, and a sense of drudgery that may eventually become an endless grey depression. It is surely significant that a recent book on stress in doctors has been given a cartoon-like cover and chapter headings, as if even doctors, or perhaps, especially doctors, must lighten the subject and make sure that any doctor observed reading the book can be considered to be doing no more than indulging in a little amusing pleasure (Haslam, 1994). Today's popular focus for stress is one that looks outside the stressed individual: to his work hours, his work conditions, or to his boss; while those who aim to help tend to focus on what the stressed person should do, adding an extra burden to his day. Both these approaches are easier than getting to grips with the pressured and driven qualities that exist in the stressed person's make-up. For instance, in a doctor there will have been imperatives that made him choose his work, and these factors can live on, demanding a way of working that pressurizes. Causative factors such as these are closer to home and more powerful than the external ones.

In this chapter I propose first to explore some of the doctor's

21

external stresses before considering possible internal ones, and finally some of the finer – though far-reaching – effects of stress.

Working with people who are ill and dying is particularly stressful. Sick people rely on those around them, not just for physical nursing, but also for psychological support. They have not the energy to cope with what is going on in their lives and so lose interest in those around them and often have a short fuse with those who care for them. But even in comparatively simple day-to-day situations they can make considerable demands. For example, this morning I was called to the house of a sixty-seven-year-old lady who had chest pain extending into her arms. At first she seemed composed as she answered my questions and she was apparently quite relaxed while I examined her. Her husband, I noticed, left us in the room, from what I supposed was consideration for his wife's privacy.

Before talking about my findings, I asked if I could fetch the lady's husband so as to talk to them both. She agreed and I went to fetch him. The doors were open and I surprised him as he stood fidgeting nervously at the window. I quickly realised his anxiety was such that he had not heard when I had tapped on the door of his room.

We went in to his wife together and I told them I felt reasonably sure she was having a heart attack, and that I wanted to send her into hospital. 'Yes,' she said, 'I thought I was.' Now her anxiety showed through as she fell over her words, looked strained, and admitted for the first time that her pain was very severe.

I gave her the necessary treatment and pain relief, made the telephone calls and wrote the letter for the hospital. Her husband phoned their daughter to ask her to come. I could not help but see how he became confused over the keypad of the telephone and had difficulty in telling his daughter about her mother's pain and probable coronary thrombosis.

The ambulance arrived and the team made their assessment. They had come quickly and at first were tense with concern for what they might have to do for the lady. I told them what I had given her and they settled to their well-known and careful work routines.

Hardly had the ambulance men put the lady in the ambulance and her husband climbed in to sit by her, when the daughter drove up. She had tears in her eyes as I put her in the picture and answered her immediate questions. She spoke briefly with her parents and made the decision to follow to the hospital in her car. I reminded her that her concentration would not be good, gently asking her to take her time driving to hospital and gave her the name of the ward.

This was a Sunday morning. It was a single early morning call, so I was in a position to observe myself in relation to that one piece of work. I had fielded the anxiety and concern of six sets of people. There was my own concern to check for signs of immediate life-threatening complications, to gain the patient's agreement to admission, to use my skills and judgement to give her an adequate dose of fast-acting intravenous pain relief and make efficient arrangements with hospital and ambulance. There was also the panic and need for information in first the patient and then her husband, with feelings of fear at the threatening unknown in her and, for him, of uselessness and a sense of an imminent threat that life might fall apart. There was the hospital doctor who, in this case, quickly accepted the need for admission but had initially shown his impatience at being disturbed first thing on a Sunday. Then there was the ambulance team: their anxiety quickly settled after they had efficiently checked out the patient's situation and requirements with me. Lastly there was the shocked daughter with her whole range of feelings that became focused as the answers to her questions enabled her to know more about what she was facing, and her anxiety as her regular life was suddenly injected with the threat of deep loss. Now all these people were balanced and kindly folk who largely carried their own feelings, and yet I was aware of the changing tone and pressure of their feelings while I was with them. I was ready for a cup of coffee when I returned home, noticeably tired by that one hour's work. Yet this is a small and normal enough part of any doctor's working day – just one patient out of the thirty or more with whom he is in contact, either face-to-face or by telephone.

Whenever a doctor is with a patient, the clinical picture will include the patient's stress at being ill. It repays the doctor to clarify all the feelings involved in these situations and to be clear as to where they belong, so as to be able to apportion them to the people concerned. He spends his working life with people who are in a crisis of one sort or another, and such people will often load him with their feelings. Often, one after another, they off-load burdensome, distressing, horrific, overwhelming feelings which they are finding too much to carry and which therefore make them deeply anxious, and they learn from seeing how the doctor survives and copes with their burden. It is remarkable the extent and nature of burdens a doctor may carry for other people in the course of just one day.

Work with people who are struggling with severe illness and death can be immensely satisfying, but it is always at considerable

23

cost. Coupled with the anxieties and anguish such people often leave with their doctor are the stresses of the medical decisions he must make and which may have grave consequences.

A British Medical Association report (1992) on doctor stress points out another, perhaps less obvious, source of major stress. This is the difficulty the doctor faces when, in the middle of dealing with a patient in the consulting room, he is asked to deal with an apparently urgent call to someone else who may be acutely ill. He must then make prioritising decisions that cannot please everyone, may well have serious consequences to the life of a patient and, one way or another, can disrupt his work for the rest of the morning, perhaps for the rest of the day.

Then there are, of course, the night calls that disturb the doctor's recovery time, and evening and weekend calls that invade his personal relaxation and recuperation. Especially annoying are the inadequate resources available in the form of insufficient doctors and nurses to cover the hours worked, resulting in his being unnecessarily overloaded and stressed, and in having the time for himself and his family eroded if he is to be dependable and complete his work. And yet, of course, when they are stressed, doctors will need more time – not less – for themselves and for relaxing with those who love and care for them.

The doctors' workload is increasing rapidly. For instance, paperwork has mushroomed, giving little benefit to patients who have no understanding of this extra load as they are given less time as the doctor attempts to compensate. Indeed there are increasing public expectations: for instance, social changes have had considerable effects, with recession increasing people's fear of losing their work and resulting in employer pressure to excel and not take time out to visit doctors. Saturday morning and out of hours' work for the doctor is therefore increased, and once this pattern is established, it is then hard to reverse. While on the one hand the doctors' workload is increasing, pressing them into working faster and making them over-tired, on the other, an attitude of patient complaint, rather than team-work, is being fostered by the politicians, and increasingly there is the threat of litigation that seems to hang like gathering clouds.

These external stresses are considerable, but there are also internal ones which are even more debilitating and yet are often overlooked because they seem so personal.

There will be all sorts of reasons why a doctor may choose his career and these will live on, sometimes making extra demands that underlie the work itself.

Before I chose medicine I had some knowledge that doctoring

would encroach on my private life but this was not a factor that weighed in the balance against the choice of medicine: on the contrary, it made me favour it. With a Protestant background and work ethic, I considered it good to choose a job that demanded a lot of me. I don't like to admit it, but at that time I had a belief that the more I did for others the better I was. Also my father was a workaholic, and to seem to criticise his behaviour by not working in the same way as him was then impossible for me.

Another relevant attitude lay in a feeling that if someone was ill, then they would get attention. I now see this as arising out of an upbringing where I had the experience of getting the most personal attention and concern when I was ill. Illness and closeness were inseparable. As a teenager looking to what I would do with my life and searching for a close intimacy, working with illness had special appeal.

These are two small examples of a doctor's 'beliefs' that, unconscious and multiplied, can be so quietly demanding, that the doctor exists in the consulting room as much for himself as for the needs of the patient. The resulting pressure is twofold. His inner impetus of unspoken motivations stress him, pulling him this way and that, and are all in addition to doing the work involved in seeing to the patients' needs.

Now let us suppose that a doctor does get what he is unknowingly seeking from the patient, that his unconscious, hidden agenda of internal, personal, pressured needs are alive in the consultation; then there would be the probability that, as his needs are satisfied by the patient, he would unconsciously require the relationship to continue. Any suggestion that he was no longer needed because the patient had improved and was now ready to go his own way could be met with vibrations from the doctor that gave the message of, 'do not go', 'do not get better', in effect, 'keep yourself ill'. If a patient succumbs to these pressures it can result in frustrating stalemate.

And many people are very sensitive to another's needs. Alice Miller has made a special study of this aspect of human behaviour (1985). She describes how, throughout their childhood, some children experience the attitude of, 'Satisfy and please me, your parent, or you are unacceptable'. 'Make us, your parents, feel good, useful and loving, or you are unacceptable to us.' And as patients often slip their doctor into the position of standing in for their parents, such past parental attitudes may then be assumed to be present in the doctor. These patients will find it difficult to leave a doctor who is dependent on their illness.

If these interlocking sets of pressures exist in the relationship between doctor and patient, they will be most unfortunate for the patient and tend to increase the doctor's work and the stress of his relationship with the patient. Lack of movement in the relationship between patient and doctor is frustrating and stressful. On the other hand, it requires maturity on the doctor's part to take delight in people's recovery and to accept the loss he then experiences as a patient walks away.

There are other stresses that result from a doctor's not being able to face some aspect of his work. A particularly prevalent one is in relation to death. A colleague feared death so much himself that he could not make rational and reasoned decisions about dying patients' needs. His patients could not rely on him to be a companion on the last leg of their life journey. He knew he feared death, but he could not himself say much more than that, and could not therefore make any inroads into understanding the fear and the stresses that death caused him.

I was to learn a lot in this respect from one of my patients. I had often visited during his wife's last prolonged illness and her death at home. Now he, too, wanted to stay at home with his own fatal illness, and for a short time I visited him regularly for his pain control. Finally he developed a complicating congestive heart failure and was clearly weakening. One afternoon he asked me if I would return after the evening surgery. I naïvely thought he was concerned about the treatment of his pain for the night and, on this assumption, agreed to return. I arrived and found that his housekeeper had been asked to prepare two dishes of a light fruit purée which were now placed near his bed beside a nice cheese and a good bottle of wine. He asked me to open the wine: I ate some cheese and we enjoyed the purée and sipped the wine together.

I had realized that those who believe they are dying will frequently need to talk over their lives as if gathering it all together in their mind's eye, being wistful here, and satisfied there; needing to run over it all, rounding it off, but also needing to hand over the summary of their lives to another. It is as if they need to be sure that what they have done is not lost, and so now this man went over his life with me in that hour we spent together. It was very moving and very real. I felt very close to him. That was the first time that anyone wished me goodbye before they died. It was as if this generous man took me by the hand and accompanied *me* on a journey right up to death. This has become a model of the experience of dying for me, something to work towards. I suspect he knew he was giving me something precious. I offer it to you and am sure he would approve. He died early in the morning. His housekeeper was with him.

26

There is intrinsically nothing to fear in death. The feeling is to do with the person who fears rather than with death. Joanna Field (1952) says she feels it is a question of whether people can accept annihilation, coupled with the fact that other people will go on without them.

If a doctor has an unspoken, unrealised and unrealistic belief that he must control illness and prevent death, then when he finds he cannot, he will have a considerable feeling of failure and guilt: both unpleasant and stressful feelings.

Alison Wertheimer (1986) suggests that it is the feeling of guilt which leads to the doctor being unable to communicate or remain with patients who are dying. Note, it is only their sense of guilt, not anything they have or have not done; but the doctor cannot look the patient in the eye nor continue to relate to those he feels he has somehow failed. Yet if both patient and doctor are on the same journey through life which inevitably ends in death, then, other things being equal, there is in reality no failure for the doctor in his patient dying. It is a right and proper thing for people to do. It is part of life.

Usually guilt in the doctor is not due to his lack of skill or the quality of the patient's treatment, but rather to his learned outlook on life. It is noteworthy that most people feel guilt after someone close to them dies, and this normal experience will occur in the doctor as well as the relatives. Both the doctor and his patients will benefit if he can free himself by understanding the factual baselessness of this guilt feeling in relation to his medical skills.

Not infrequently, the relative of a patient who has died will make complaints. It is perhaps natural enough that they complain somehow, or somewhere, if we consider that they must now face the daunting distress of deep loss and the pain of separation. In my experience, complaints happen most frequently when the relative has come rather late onto the scene and, no doubt partly as a result of this, has not moved very far along the journey of acceptance. Those who have been present and lived through the various phases of the experience will have moved on from that point. They are past the stage when defensive blaming occurs, and into a far more sensitive phase of sharing and involvement. Frequently the doctor will be included in this tightly formed, warm group. For its members it is, to say the least, painful and stressful to suddenly be drawn out of this closer way of relating and into one where there is little or no appreciation, but rather, complaint or outright blame. The relative who arrives belatedly (and who is just beginning to experience his loss of the loved one), and who now discovers himself left outside a group of this nature, may also find himself particularly sensitive to feelings of exclusion. Jealousy of an outsider may therefore lie behind his complaint. When this is thought to be the dynamic, the sooner a doctor separates from the family group, leaving its members to sort themselves out, the faster will the force of complaint die away. The family need is for all its members to be involved together.

Just as doctors may have a personal need to control physical pain and prevent death, so they often carry an inner need to control psychological pain, distress and anxiety.

The first time I referred a patient to a psychiatrist I expected that the patient would somehow take the suggestion as a slight or as an insult. Similarly a colleague once confided in me that when a member of his family needed psychiatric help, he experienced a sense of shock that other people had seen this as quite all right and as something that could be talked about and handled just like any other aspect of life. As a result he now became able to free himself from a considerable fear of mental distress.

In Victorian England mental illness was put away out of sight, locked in castle-like buildings hidden behind trees. Today lesser disturbances of the person are glossed over with knowing smiles and talk of a 'colourful personality', or other 'positive' descriptions of people being 'real characters'. Deep in society there is concern to cover up mental anguish and distress, to discount it and pretend it is not there.

I suspect that in my own case this developed from some fear of breaking-up, from a sense of collapse, of non-functioning, being out of control, aimlessness, non-contactability, being irrational, the fear that others would find me not worth troubling with, that I would be passed by on the other side, or that I might be seen to have such strange emotions that they might destroy others or at least be seen as potentially dangerous.

This is important in understanding patients. Stress-producing beliefs can be powerful, and each patient will have his own versions. Their power is dissipated by pin-pointing the fears and talking about them. The doctor cannot make contact with the reality of the patient's inner world unless he can make and name a diagnosis in their feeling areas and talk openly with the patient about it. Unless he can do this, the patient remains locked into his condition; locked into unknowing with no signpost showing the ways out; locked into an impotent inability to work them through. Similarly, the doctor has the frustration of feeling he is not enabling the patient to move on.

Nevertheless, doing this can be difficult. Take for example a widow of some years' standing, who is unhappy and distraught and yet not clear in herself why. As she talks, the doctor perceives her loneliness. 'What do you do about your very real loneliness, Mrs Smith?' There is a sudden visible sense of shock that leaps up in her face and the doctor is acutely aware of her pain. It is so easy for him to view this as caused by his own clumsiness so that he decides to hold his tongue another time. But that would be to protect the doctor from his painful realization of her need to scream, whereas for her, her distress is at last seen for what it is and brought out into the open where it can be shared. Her loneliness was there already; the doctor has not caused it. He is saying, 'I know and I am here with you'. First comes the diagnosis, the doctor's recognition of the very real feeling of loneliness in the patient; then it is spoken, so that it can be perceived and sampled. The two of them can then mull over its breadth and depth. It can be owned by the patient, so that she is at last freed to seek to do something about it. And it is worth noting that this has a positive, ongoing, freeing effect – quite the reverse of protective behaviour by the doctor. There is also an economy of effort for patient and doctor, and the doctor is freed from a sense of responsibility with its consequent stress – but only if he can face the patient's feelings and relax any tendency to attempt their control.

It is remarkable how little literature there is on this subject of internal stress in doctors although doctors seem free with their observations on their patients. Dr W. D. K. Johnson ploughs a lonely furrow when he reviews the psychological literature on the subject (1991). He then goes on to point out that doctors are frequently withdrawn from emotion, and that their need for a sense of professional success with patients limits their capacity for emotional intimacy, which in turn limits support from friends and family. With reduced support a doctor is more easily toppled into depression, alcohol and drug abuse, or suicide.

It can easily be forgotten that the individual doctor may have his own particular difficulties so that his work will take more out of him than from others. One or other of the following is likely to occur in most doctor's lives, but doctors themselves often prefer to forget these factors. It should be obvious that pain or ongoing discomfort from back trouble will sap his strength; or that the inevitable phases of major adjustments in a doctor's marriage will use up considerable emotional energy; or that when children are small and very demanding a doctor who is also a parent will be chronically short on sleep; or when his elderly relative passes through a phase of increasing weakness and dependency, a doctor's stamina for his work will be depleted; or when a parent eventually dies his energy will largely be taken up with grieving and internal adjustments. Also it is common now for a doctor to have a spouse who is in full-time professional work. There is then often little leeway within the family for that doctor to receive extra support and understanding at home when, as inevitably sometimes happens, the doctor is unduly stressed by work. When a doctor, for whatever reason, is under the weather he may shut off and isolate himself for his own self-preservation, or his current experience may so mirror the patient's condition that the doctor becomes overly empathetic with the patient's circumstances. It is as if, when doctors are ill, they have no energy to maintain the boundaries of their own person, so that the patient's situation can seem to mingle with his own. Ill and stressed doctors are therefore particularly vulnerable to their patients' feelings and, while his strength is low and his energy and flexibility reduced by his own personal needs, his skills will not be so available for dealing with patients. The already stressed or ill doctor, therefore, easily becomes further stressed and wearied. It is as if his personal boundaries are blurred and other people have more ready access into his being. The doctor does well to acknowledge this and give high priority to taking care of himself and maintaining the boundaries of his personality.

A partnership must be human enough to be flexible in these situations, or the doctors in the practice will lose their sensitivity to patients. But there are less obvious factors too; for instance, we are told that a high proportion of dyslexic people take up medicine as a career. The increased concentration and effort these people must put into verbal communication is considerable and will disproportionately deplete their finite energy resources. Or again, a doctor who can and does communicate at depth may well be more wearied by his work than someone else who works at a more superficial level. All ways of working are valuable, and different ways of working are needed in the population a practice serves; therefore the resulting effects on each individual doctor of the different skills and methods they use need similar acceptance, and to be respected by a doctor's partners. Often, however, doctors instead mete out numerical work comparisons and other pressures which are dehumanising and only increase the stress for all of them.

Sometimes, however, doctors become patients themselves. Over the years it has intrigued me to see how difficult it is for doctors to allow themselves to go to a colleague for good family doctor care. There are peripheral issues here, such as, that it will take time, or hesitation over bothering a colleague with something the doctor surely knows how to deal with himself, or perhaps there is some alarm that the other doctor will do the job better than he can. Yet it is more than these. If a dominant need to control physical and psychological pain has driven a person into becoming a doctor, his need to be in control will probably lead to difficulty in trusting others with his own pain. He therefore keeps away from his own doctor and, incidentally, from the focus of another's concern that might enable him to review his attitudes and gain relief from his psychological distress.

Two situations from my past come to mind with regard to this need for control. As a young house-surgeon in hospital I needed a minor operation. I was pleased my consultant would do it: I could choose the timing and I would be on familiar ground and with people I had grown to trust deeply. That morning we did the ward round, and then I presented myself to the ward sister who showed me my bed. 'Get undressed, put on this gown and hop into bed.' All familiar enough. I undressed and put on the gown. Then I thought I would pull back the curtains before hopping into bed. I pulled them back, and as I did so was hit with a sense of nakedness, not at all limited to the physical: where was my white coat, my cloak against illness?

Here was a sharp transition from being a knowing doctor in control of illness (as he thought), to being a patient soon to be cut about by someone else. I was subdued and shaken and, the day after my small operation, pleased to slip out of the ward and go on my pre-arranged holiday, happy to leave behind a part of life that had no place in my preferred image of myself.

For patients, hospitals are places of illness, disability and death; of recognising the limitations which their bodies place on life, and the loss that must be followed by the pain of grieving. For me, there had been a glossing over of these by considering hospitals as places filled only with the excitement of training, of mind over matter, of 'miracles' resulting from an accumulation of controlling knowledge, and an assumption of power over death.

The other situation which comes to mind relates to visits to my doctor. I had been to doctors for vaccinations and inoculations, and for some injury to a joint. I made these visits to prepare for going abroad or as the result of games of rugger; all good, healthy, active stuff. I could, and I did, regard them as normal. More recently, however, I have found myself having neck trouble with pressure on the nerves to my arms which has affected my work, my sleep and many other activities. My doctor had me undress and he put my neck and arms through their movements, touching and feeling and examining with his hands, at the same time asking the sort of

31

questions I knew about. But now they were about *me* and *my* body. The combination of talk and touch was soothing. I was being cared for. I was allowing myself to be cared for. I was experiencing something I had not allowed myself to experience when I had doctored myself. I was discovering what patients going to their doctors experience. I was no longer having to carry the burden of it on my own and I relaxed. My defences about my condition began to slide away. The symptoms could be better defined now, and I discovered those symptoms had been around longer than I had cared to think. I had let myself believe them to be 'tennis elbow', although there had been no confirmatory tenderness. It was as if I had needed the support of another to allow me to see the extent of the trouble. There then followed the hypotheses, the plan of investigation to narrow down to a diagnosis, and a survey of the possible lines of treatment with their likelihood of usefulness. From keeping illness at a distance and in a fog of surrounding anxieties about how big it might all be and of how incapacitating it might become, things had changed. My condition was now real: I knew what it was and where it might actually go. This allowed me to get on with life: the illness had changed from the realm of flights of fancy to a reality that, while unpleasant, was possible to face.

These are examples of uncovering the defence of control which I had to illness and which in turn will have added to the stress levels of my work as a doctor. No doubt all doctors have their own brands of defence.

So far this chapter has been about the causative factors of a doctor's stresses: both those which are external to the doctor and which he meets as a result of dealing with people who are ill and anxious, and those which result from his own individuality and unconsciously held attitudes. In general, in society, attitudinal stress is increasing as society focuses more on money and loses sight of life's other valuable assets and, while stress is not itself an illness, too much of it can be so debilitating that it destroys health. What then of the effects of stress?

One general and more obvious result of an ever-increasing work load is less private time with family and friends – even to the extent of being stressed past the point where the doctor is able to use his remaining private time to make effective contact with loved ones. Professor Robert Lane (1993) points out that the one most important factor in producing a sense of well-being is the security of relationships in the home. The stress of excessive workload therefore cuts right to the heart of the doctor's well-being and can draw him into a vicious downward spiral.

There have been two periods in my adult life when I have

stepped away from the immediate role of doctor. On both occasions I have been delighted by what has happened inside me. The first was a year spent teaching family practice in Canada. I was suddenly in a different country, a rich mix of culture, a change in friends and a new range of small groups in the medical school with their interesting group dynamics, but there was also an intense loneliness because I was away from family and home. Alongside the excitement, there were stresses of a new kind, but they were my own and not generated by other people. I was not experiencing the tiredness of disturbed nights, the demands made by being the first person to meet whatever problem walked in off the street or called down the telephone. Released from being used as a dumping ground for the unwanted feelings of the distressed, the anxious, the depressed, and the confused, I became aware of myself in a new and exciting way.

For instance, in that university setting my days were very varied and would frequently necessitate getting up at widely different times. If, before I went to bed, I had thought out what time I needed to get up the next morning then, even if that was very early, I would wake at that time. Or again, I became aware that my memory for the ever-changing programme of work, scattered as it was in a variety of different hospitals in the town, became certain, and my internal reminder system began to give me the nudge. Time management became second nature so that I easily had the time I needed, for example, to prepare some talk for a special event; it was as if my time organisation became automatic and reliable. Then again, there was an awareness of beauty and people that both thrilled and amazed me. I had energy to listen to any kind of music and let it take me where the composer intended, whereas when stressed, I must choose music to suit my mood, because I have no energy or ability to let it affect me.

In the first chapter I referred to linear and circular thinking. Some people, I believe, become linear thinkers or never develop the ability to be circular thinkers, probably as a result of stress and a consequently high defence level. These people engage in exclusively logical thought. The ability to let the mind range out and discover whatever is there requires a stillness. The poet, John Keats, wrote of 'negative potential, a capability to be in uncertainty, mystery and doubt, without any irritable reaching after fact and reason' (1817). Wilfred Bion (1974) spoke of an ability to allow such total nothingness of intent that the smallest and weakest light can catch the attention in the still darkness of the mind. Such wonderful, unpressured awareness to one's inner self, followed by a meandering of the mind that circles and wheels so that one thought is then found to be approached from a second or third direction, result in 'Ah-ha!' experiences of linkage, and of things falling into place. Delightfully creative experiences such as these are driven out by stress and inner pressure for control.

During my year's sabbatical my awareness increased in ways like these, so that pleasure in whatever went on inside and around me multiplied. I had time for me. It felt good, exciting and whole. I felt nurtured and affirmed.

The second time I stepped out of the stress of general practice was to take two months to begin writing this book. Again I experienced the same feelings and discovered those same abilities. Previously I had considered it to have been Canada that somehow had this effect on me. I had mused that perhaps the sparsely populated northern spaciousness and the immigrant's concern for independence had something to do with it. Experiencing it again in England in this recent short break, I now see it as the result of reduced stress levels.

These enriching aspects of life are lost if stress is denied, so that consequent adjustments cannot be made. Yet many do deny stress. I remember a hospital colleague talking of a young doctor's job and saying that it was not stressful. Work, he stated, had not been extra busy of late and no one had been on holiday to make the team short-handed. Stress was not a problem, he said. That the young doctor was doing far more than a conventional full day's work, was on call at night and had dealt with a spate of deaths and the newly dead's relations, was brushed aside. Stress was being denied, presumably because that doctor could not admit it in himself.

One colleague in particular has admitted and shared his stress in his work with me. While I hope I listened and supported him, at the same time I thought, 'Why doesn't my friend sort himself out and find a way to relate to people while keeping himself separate? Why can't he live in the present without such strong anxiety about the future or guilt about the past? Why isn't he prepared to say "no" to patients?' I had made stress out to be his 'fault' rather than seeing it as a mutual problem, one that affected me just as deeply.

Year after year in case discussion groups, different doctors have spoken of their sheer distress, first expressed by the more daring member of the group, at death and dying, at grief and loss, and at the defensive attitudes of fellow staff to these same experiences, which prevented closer and more sustaining relations with those colleagues. These combine with the overload of work to crush their vitality. I hope I have heard, understood and facilitated their expression of feeling, and yet it was not until I was preparing for this book at the age of fifty-five that I was really willing to feel the sheer weight of the work myself, the lowness of spirit of an evening, the stress and tiredness that others' problems produce, and admit them in myself alongside my interest, enthusiasm and love for what I do.

I think I would have enjoyed and been interested in the human dynamics of relationships anyway, but I now see that the effort and time I have put into understanding them has also been to protect myself. That effort has been considerable. I did not let myself admit that I had to do it just to exist; so I have denied my stress in order to avoid seeing it or admitting it in myself, locking it in and making me less able to make adjustments and less free to be myself.

This narrowing of the field of vision under stress is interesting. It is as if a stressed man becomes blinkered. All the enjoyment of seeing trees and flowers, the sun and play of light, the children playing and the welcoming smiles of people as they pass, are lost. The warmth and companionship of life is no longer available to the stressed person. What a loss this is to all life's carers, who need for themselves the same care they give to others. How sterile life can become. Not only is the stressed doctor losing out on the sustenance of the wider view but also he cannot see the breadth and depth of the situations he works with, and therefore even his ability to take care of patients will be reduced. His defences are raised to the point of blinding him to all but what lies in the narrow focus of his distressed mind and, sensing his reduced ability, he loses a feeling of satisfaction for work well done.

Stress affects the doctor's work, his interests, his relationships with family and friends and his ability to receive sustenance and recharge himself. At the beginning of this chapter it was observed that stress can be a potential, or even actual, killer when, for example, it reduces awareness in a car driver so that he makes critical errors of judgement. But stress is a killer in so many other ways: it kills relationships both at work and at home, and kills the spirit of a man so that life is barren, sometimes even to the point of making him contemplate suicide.

It may be useful for a doctor to conceive an image of himself, for instance, as if he were a glass partly full of water. Sometimes he will see the glass as being half empty and acutely aware of the emptiness, feel sad, so that the water itself may seem to have lost its sparkle. At other times he can choose to move his focus and take a delight in seeing that his glass is half full, realising that he can drink deeply from it and knowing that he can later work to refill his glass; he can be excited by planning its filling and in the knowledge that there is enjoyment in the task. Some such picture can give a doctor freedom to value his whole self, to be aware of all his varied emotions and be alive to and take due pleasure in all his senses, taking care to sample and value both his life's emptiness and its fullness.

Work on stress relief must surely be given conscious priority by family doctors, but it needs to be personal in the doctor before he can really deal with it at any depth in others. It is rightly a major focus for his understanding. Can the doctor allow himself to see himself as a person just like his patients and take that first step of acknowledging stress in himself? Can he admit his own need for care and as a result be able to sample life at a satisfying depth? Can he monitor and learn about his own stressful reactions to life and take the road to a fuller, more aware and satisfying life for himself, for his family and – by extension – for his patients?

CHAPTER 4

Out of Hours' Work and Visits

Probably nothing encroaches and intrudes into the doctor's personal life more clearly and obviously than his work when he is 'on call'. It is a major source of his stress. He will have worked a full week but is then still at the beck and call of people who feel they cannot wait until office hours come round again. In the United Kingdom he has a responsibility twenty-four hours a day, seven days a week and three hundred and sixty-five days a year, a heavy commitment by all accounts. He may make reciprocal arrangements to share the out of hours' work with partners or neighbouring practices, but that arrangement brings more concentrated work and responsibility during the hours he is on duty and 'paying them back', and in any case his work hours remain too long. Being 'on call' entails disturbance to sleep patterns and makes the days that follow ones of tiredness and struggle while reducing recuperative and recreational time. Doctors, like everyone else, need time for themselves but they need it more especially because ill people are a particularly heavy burden. As a result it is essential that they put time and energy into preserving personal time for themselves.

The last chapter referred to some doctors' denial of stress. It is especially a characteristic of younger people. As a student I lived some years in a student hostel on Commercial Road, in east London. The hostel rooms all overlooked the cobbled road which was a main route to and from the London docks and so carried a large number of lorries. Many of the lorry drivers made the journey at night when they were not held up by daytime traffic, and the intermittent nighttime noise of planks or chains bouncing about on the back of empty lorries as they passed over the rough road frequently disturbed our sleep. We used to say we were used to it and that it did not affect us, and yet in our more honest moments we would admit that in the holidays and away from that road, we would get off to sleep faster, sleep less fitfully, feel far brighter and have more energy. No doubt, feeling better was not all due to the reduced noise disturbance, but when talking more intimately in twos or threes, we would admit that disturbance due to noise was a major factor in tiring and stressing us with its invidious cumulative effect. It is strange that such external factors are so often denied as a cause of stress. The truth is that recurrent disturbance of sleep is immensely debilitating: at its extreme it is effectively used as a form of torture to disorientate a prisoner under interrogation. Its denial then is perhaps a part of youth's preferred belief that, for them, all things are possible. Stress, from whatever cause, is often similarly denied.

Frequently a doctor's own self-image seems founded on an unspoken belief that he must be above any feelings that might be seen as weakness. It is as if he feels that doctors would not be good doctors if they were to admit these feelings, as if this would mean the fulfilment of their role would be blemished and they could not then be trusted to put their patients first. Many, however, then put patients not only first, but also second, third and fourth until they themselves, as well as their families, are relegated right off the bottom of the priority list. These attitudes can have serious consequences in depleting the doctor's resources. He may ruin his own, and his family's lives, while patients with similar attitudes will gravitate to him because they affirm each other in their attitudes, each making it unlikely for the other to be critical – a first step in the process of change.

Now that I am older, I am more aware of my needs and the effects of stress on me. My available energy is less, so that I am more often aware that my reserves are low and of what drains them. At the same time I seem to have less concern for any apparent loss of face, so that I am willing to admit my energy depletion. It is remarkably freeing as by admitting the effects while I experience them more, I can also work to make them more acceptable.

Dr Fleur Fisher of the British Medical Association has argued that until doctors themselves begin to see the admission of stress as a sign of strength, the inadequate human resources given to medical care in the face of the ever-increasing expectations of society is unlikely to be adjusted accordingly (1992). There is so often a bluff in doctors' denial, as if they must appear completely in control and be capable of offering a totally safe responsibility. Perhaps it is difficult for them to admit their stress to themselves or even to countenance it in colleagues, when stressed patients produce so much work and are sometimes the butt of scorn and jokes. However, only when such stress is admitted can the doctor make changes in his life so as to ease it, or negotiate with partners for adjustments, or openly lay it on the political table to claim the need for contractual changes as began to happen in 1993 and 1994.

Why are so many doctors apparently happy to take on excessively heavy burdens of work spread over such long hours? Sometimes a doctor can feel so burdened with a patient's distress that he feels the condition must be too much for the patient to bear. He may then slip into attempting to protect the patient and try to remove the distress by excess visiting and care. As both patient and doctor need to be responsible for themselves, it would be better for the doctor to learn to handle his own distress, leaving patients to handle theirs. What is clear, however, is that a doctor's attitudes have major effects as stress factors.

You may know *A Fortunate Man*, by John Berger, a book which is illustrated with many evocative photos by Jean Mohr (Berger, 1976). It describes some weeks spent observing and talking with a country doctor as he went about his work. At first sight it gives a warm picture of caring and concern with the photos increasing the feeling of sensitivity, so that when I read it, I was impressed by the degree of care those patients received, and yet, at a different level, it filled me with distress for the doctor. He was working, working, working, and this attitude to his work seemed to be encouraged by the book. It was as if he saw his worth as deriving more from what he did than from the person he was. I was left wondering if this had been relevant to his later suicide.

Many doctors are workaholics, dependent on their work. To my mind the central question that lies behind the workaholic approach is, 'From where does the individual get his value?' Childhood development theory may offer some insight. Imagine a mother with her baby: she plays with it, talks to it and repeatedly gives the message: 'I like you. I enjoy you. Whatever you do, I love you.' Through repeated and consistent experiences like this, the baby grows up with a sense of inherent value and worth, but as he gets older he begins to do things. To his sense of intrinsic value is now added the understanding that he has also made a fun sandcastle, or helped mother by carrying some shopping today, or whatever else it was he did. Doing this something was an extra. It was not necessary for his sense of feeling valuable and worthwhile, but gave added value. Workaholics often seem to work to give themselves value, rather than added value. Presumably it covers up a sense of emptiness or guilt. I do not know how such people grow old gracefully, able to sit on a seat in the sun by their door and contemplate their eighty years – and yet their ageing bodies will demand that change. People must find their value in what they *are*.

I remember a doctor who regularly did more than thirty home visits in a week, and that was in addition to the weekends and the nights when he was on call. I admired his energy, but was concerned for him. What drove him on? As I got to know him more it seemed to me that it was his need to please (upon which depended his ability to feel good about himself) which dictated his visiting, rather than the real needs of his patients.

Some patients were actually disturbed by his visits. One man came to me saying, 'I am worried. I have seen my regular doctor who has checked things through for me and I believed I knew what was going on in my body. I'm doing all the right things to stay as well as possible, but that other doctor keeps visiting me. I regularly get out and about, so he must be doing this because he knows something I don't. I must have some serious illness that I'm not being told about by my doctors. What do I do to find out?' The doctor's own personal anxiety and confusion in this situation was, I think, diffusing into the patient who, not knowing the cause of the doctor's anxiety, started jumping to conclusions.

A doctor does not help people advance their development if he cannot make a similar journey himself. I really had to address my own workaholism, or at least start to progress through to understanding it. Personal changes like these free the doctor to make realistic decisions about his work patterns, and unobtrusively have a beneficial effect on patients and practice staff.

The quantity of out of hours' work is steadily rising. In 1994 the government's own figures showed that night visits had multiplied by five in the previous twenty-five years and doubled in the last three. This represents a huge increase in individual doctor disturbance and stress. It demands change in the way doctors work and, as a result, family practices in more populated areas are now once more experimenting with forming doctor co-operatives. A local co-operative formed recently to share the out of hours' emergency cover of their patients has made a lot of difference to the doctors. One of them has pointed out that the less frequent on-call duties, although heavier, have enabled him to be certain about when his time is his own and when it is committed to patients. It has removed the sense of confusion and resentment that so often develops when time for private life is excessively restricted. However, co-operatives mean that a consistent attitude by the personnel involved in out of hours' work will be lost; a consistency which, over time, educates patients as to what is a reasonable expectation given the restricted resources of the service. I am sure that very soon co-operatives and similar arrangements will have the overall effect of trivialising the out of hours calls, unnecessarily increasing the spread of medical work into the night. Also, of course, co-operatives are only a different way for doctors to pack excess work into their lives.

Dr Knox reports a study where a practice visiting rate was reduced by over 40 per cent by introducing a system where there was telephone discussion between doctor and patient before requests for visits were accepted (1989). That is a reduction of over one-third. The doctor is more free to function effectively if not overwhelmed with unnecessary home visits. It is clear therefore that changes in approaches to work can make major differences.

How can the doctor approach his out of hours' work so as to be effective and yet keep his commitment to reasonable proportions? Most young doctors in training want to sort out their doctor's bag, check their emergency drugs to see that they have everything they may need, make sure that their car is reliable and arrange to have a telephone by the bed. Attention to details such as these can make a lot of difference. But there are also different ways of handling patients. Basically a doctor is dealing with two things in the patient: one is a concern for the clinical condition (the patient perceiving himself as being in a life-threatening situation or in unnecessary discomfort) and the other is the patient's anxiety. Usually there will be both, and the doctor, as well as his patient, will be rewarded if he is prepared to deal with both.

While both of these exist in the patient, they are mirrored in the doctor. Does he have the knowledge and skill to deal with the physical problems and can he deal with his own anxiety and distress at the patient's situation? There are four areas that need attention, two in the patient and the two mirrored in the doctor.

Erik Erikson, in his intriguing book on personal and society's development, *Childhood and Society* (1977), makes a distinction between different levels of anxiety. I will use the words 'concern' and 'anxiety' to denote different levels. He points out that infants can do nothing about many of their concerns and therefore, without the rational and able parent present to adjust things imaginatively for it, its concerns may develop, increasing through anxiety, to an anxiety that knows no bounds, into panic. In adults, on the other hand, concern is something that can be understood and analysed, and adjustments made. They have an ability to prevent concerns from becoming so great as to tip over into incapacitating anxiety. This picture of a developing ability is helpful both for the doctor's understanding of himself and for his approach to anxious patients. Every adult patient has been an infant and has had the experience of diffuse anxiety that can magnify and even produce an illusion of danger where none really exists. So long as the danger remains illusory, the anxieties have no avenue for mastery or escape. Adults will therefore have reminiscent experiences reflecting infantile impotence and numbing anxiety. A current experience can flip them back into feelings from the past, and this is especially likely to occur when circumstances force them back into a child-like dependency and vulnerability. The feeling of being ill is just such a circumstance, so that people facing illness are vulnerable to anxiety on a variety of counts. Patients need to work through their feelings to find their new reality, but they will often turn urgently to the doctor while in this state of mind, as if to a surrogate parent. Exploring the patient's perspective or inner world is especially helpful when attempting to relieve their anxiety.

There is another practical factor of particular importance in family medicine. In medical school training, young doctors learn to listen, check out with questions, examine, hypothesize, test, diagnose and treat. As beds in hospital are a scarce resource, this is all done immediately or planned as soon as possible. In family practice, conditions are different and there is an extra step to consider. Here the doctor listens, checks out with questions, examines and then makes an extra decision: is it appropriate for this patient's condition and frame of mind to attempt to work the problem through immediately and totally? Is it necessary, or even preferable, to go down an urgent line of investigation or treatment, or is the prognosis and patient need such that it can – and often should – be put on hold? (Of course it must be possibile to move the patient from one grouping to the other, from non-urgent to urgent, as the situation unfolds.) Patients themselves need time to take in and adjust to their new condition. In family practice doctors are used to giving this time and must often see the patient again to aid the process. If the illness is not life-threatening, time must be given anyway, and such time can also be taken over the detail of diagnosis and treatment, both for medical reasons and for the sake of the psyche.

When a doctor is on emergency call outside regular work hours, and is first contacted by telephone, this extra step is even more appropriate as he must also work to preserve his own recuperative time. He needs to firmly hold the concept that he is only on call to urgent and necessary situations and to work to a point where the patient is safe and as comfortable as possible. This is a right management issue. Listen; question the patient over the telephone to clarify the condition; then if – still without seeing and examining the patient – the doctor can exclude serious conditions likely to deteriorate or cause relievable discomfort, then there only remains the task of dealing with the patient's anxiety. If that, too, can be reasonably relieved on the telephone, no visit is necessary. The patient can be seen in normal working hours to sort things further, and can be invited meanwhile to phone again if symptoms change. All these steps can frequently be undertaken safely over the telephone. Patients usually find this appropriate because their anxiety is eased by learning of the reality of their condition. It does mean, however, that the doctor must be ready and willing to control his own anxiety without feeling compelled to visit as his only way of allaying it.

Here then is a structure that can reduce visiting levels while still enabling a doctor to do a safe and effective job. It results in his being less tired and more able to do his work the following day – to everyone's greater comfort. He can develop these skills and abilities. A useful exercise is to record telephone contacts for later review and exploration of options, and so evolve new telephone skills.

Turning now to the stresses of the job itself, it is my belief that off-loading feeling is especially powerful over the telephone. Certainly it has been for me, and my observations of other doctors suggest it is frequently so for them. It must surely be because the usual visual ways of assessing anxiety levels and of calming people are not available. The geographical separation of the people involved acts as a barrier but, be that as it may, it would explain why so frequently doctors cannot allow themselves to use the telephone to both the patient's and their own best advantage, and merely accept patients' requests without any real discussion.

However, a careful focus on telephone skills enables this difficulty to be converted into an advantage. As anxiety is uncomfortable, then reducing the patient's anxiety will also reduce the anxiety he may off-load onto the doctor holding the telephone at home. This direct, unconscious communication from the patient can be used by the doctor to monitor what is going on in a patient. Monitoring the level of the anxiety the doctor experiences can become a sure indicator of the patient's anxiety level. It is important, therefore, for the doctor to analyse his feelings. If it is his own anxiety, arising in response to the clinical material he is hearing, then he needs to go and visit; if it is the patient's, he knows the patient is anxious (even without the ability to confirm it with visual observations) and he needs to understand that anxiety. For instance, it may be that there is something the doctor still does not know, so he must investigate further. When he is confident that factual communication has been good and that there are no more anxiety-producing patient concerns to uncover, then he works to reduce the patient's anxiety. If he can reduce it, the anxiety he has been carrying for the patient will also diminish and the conversation can end with both being relaxed and at ease. If in the end he is not at ease, then I suggest he visit the patient. In this case, however, the doctor has the advantage of knowing the detail of what he will be facing and much of the necessary talking will already have been done.

There are numerous other ways of easing anxiety and each doctor can discover his own once he has seen the need for it. In the past, relatives were given something to do, like fetching 'Hot water please and plenty of it.' Relatives often feel anxious at their impotence in the face of illness. Some reasoned activity can therefore be suggested and relatives be requested to phone again if things are not improving. This invitation can in itself be very reassuring: it reminds the patient that the doctor remains interested and if necessary is there to help further. Newly-weds, for instance, may never have been alone with the responsibility of looking after someone who is ill. That the doctor is willing for them to contact him if they develop further concerns is eminently reassuring.

In this regard, the fact that the patient has already spoken to the doctor is calming. If he has not rebutted their concern, but has listened, and his questions and interest have been obvious and full, their anxiety to be understood and heard will dissipate. Even clinical concerns, which may be minor as the doctor understands them, can hold major anxiety for the patient but, once explored by their doctor, can assume their rightful proportion.

There are various useful approaches when on call and on the telephone. For instance: 'What have you tried already, Mr Smith? I would like you to try X, Y or Z.' Explain why it may be useful and ask him to phone again in an hour or so if things are not improving. Often, the fact that the patient has disencumbered himself of much of his anxiety by being in touch by telephone, and that the doctor has let him know that it is not the feared cancer or some rampant infection or whatever, will have improved the situation considerably. Similarly, the home remedy the doctor has suggested may also have been very effective. If, on the other hand, there has been no change in the hour, nothing is lost; the doctor now needs to visit because the patient's concern has remained and he needs to deal with it in person. Now, however, it is the doctor who has decided that he must go.

I find it helps considerably to remind myself that whoever telephones is asking for help for *their* problem. Some people seem to have the attitude that it is the doctor's problem. This is wrong. The doctor is there, in the first instance, to advise the patient about their problem; doing anything more is optional.

It also helps considerably to talk to the person who is ill. This can only be a general guide but it is often possible when a third party rings for the telephone to be handed over to the patient. The doctor can then listen and question the patient directly, and so deal with the individual anxieties of the ill person. It may then be necessary to speak to the relative if they share the patient's anxiety or are the source of a quite different anxiety.

Good use of the telephone may save the need for a visit but, more importantly, it can be very effective in patient care. It may, for instance, enable a doctor to advise calling the ambulance immediately, or give advice as to what to do while they await the doctor's arrival (such as to sit the patient up with legs down in acute left ventricular failure). Clearly it enables the doctor to judge the urgency, and so more accurately to prioritise his work. Therefore in some cases it may be life-saving to talk the situation through on the telephone as soon as a call comes in.

There is a further spin-off to the doctor discussing visits before setting off. All doctors have experienced situations where they have felt manipulated and set off to make a visit feeling annoyed. Many tell me this happens quite frequently. When it happens to me I find myself burning considerable energy in disgruntled, irritated feelings. I find this tiring and occasionally it can spoil the rest of the day. By talking through the patient's problem on the telephone first, I find this happens far less. It is partly that I do fewer visits but also because, when I have obtained the information about the patient first, my clinical interest or concern has been aroused, which means that I want to go, rather than feeling that I am being manipulated by some unfortunate behaviour. I also find that when I know the details already, I have time to adjust to what I am likely to meet as I travel to the visit. It is much easier on myself and far more comfortable.

But work to reduce patient anxiety needs to begin long before the telephone is picked up. Focusing on anxiety during routine daytime consultations will reduce out of hours' telephone calls and visits. Most doctors feel that this is likely considering that an anxious patient will not easily relax in the evenings or get off to sleep. There are various indicators to support this belief. For instance, there is an increased patient contact rate when a new, inexperienced doctor comes into the practice; there is the noticeable increase in a community's or society's anxiety during unsettled conditions such as financial recession, very unseasonal and extreme weather and after major accidents or national disasters – in other words, when people are forced to question their own safety. A settled partnership has noticeably more settled and less anxious patients. It is expedient for a practice not to make fast, unplanned or mammoth changes, and to keep patients well-informed whenever changes must be made. Practice newsletters or, at times of major change, open practice meetings are very beneficial in this regard, and practice Patient Participation Groups (Pritchard, 1993) play an ongoing, calming role in the community. Good listening skills on the part of the doctor enable patients to feel their concerns will be taken into account.

An example of work undertaken in a consultation to produce a settled, less anxious patient is as follows. People come for consultations to discuss their situation. If it is an acute problem, the doctor may be seeing them at the end of the day and he talks through their problem. He explores with the patient the options and, if appropriate, initiates their chosen treatment. Many people will then go home still feeling anxiety for the night or the weekend ahead. 'What if it gets worse?' 'When do I need to call again if things seem different?' Patients who telephone out of hours' will sometimes preface their call by saying, 'I do not want to disturb you in the night' or 'at the weekend', with the implied words 'so I am calling you now'. This reservoir of anxiety about disturbing the doctor adds to the pressure the patient or relative is dealing with, and will often tip them over into telephoning for a visit. At the end of a consultation people's tight faces relax and they become really at ease if the doctor says something like, 'Much of medicine is "Try it and see". I am on call tonight, and I want you to ring and tell me if you are concerned. We can talk about it and if I am worried, I will want to see you and we can make arrangements to meet. If I am not, then you will be able to relax when you have told me what is happening.' I could name the date on which I stumbled to this and am absolutely clear that, although apparently laying myself open to be called more often, the number of calls I received went down and not up. Above all, patient anxiety will fall if they are confident that they can make contact when they have a real need, and feel that their concerns will be heard and properly considered.

Doctors really do need to work out what is a reasonable service for patients (Middleton, 1991). It is reasonable to visit adults too incommoded to travel to the doctor's surgery for instance, but the doctor needs to portray the message in his actions that the patient is expected to get better – if that is indeed the case. 'Next time, perhaps you will come and see me at the surgery.' The doctor needs to emphasise that visits take up a great deal of his time and energy. 'Please phone me next week and tell me how this treatment is working and we will see if we need to make an appointment.'

Now whenever there is change in the air there will be resistant attitudes to it, both internally in the doctor himself and from his partners, the practice staff and patients. Everybody is made temporarily and uncomfortably more anxious by change. This anxiety results in pressure on the individual to continue working in the group's settled, and therefore preferred, way rather than in a new, discussed and more currently appropriate way. But things can be changed given care, discussion time and consideration of motivations.

There are all sorts of other small ways that each make for an easier, less stressful and therefore more effective way of working. For instance, the doctor on call can ask: 'Is your house number on the gate or door?' 'What colour is your house painted?' 'Will you please put on your outside light, or your car's side lights in the drive' and so forth.

In lighter vein, I remember a doctor who did prepare for ease of finding the right place in just this fashion. The patient had severe back trouble and was confined to her bed. She told the doctor to walk straight in and her bedroom was opposite the top of the stairs. He was all set for a quick entry, even to the right room in the house.

Now in such circumstances I find myself calling out something like: 'Hello, it's the doctor here' and generally making sure people know I'm coming. This doctor, however, walked unannounced straight into the bedroom, only to find a couple deeply engrossed in making love on the bed. Both heads swung around to look at him as he stood in the door with his little black bag. My friend eventually found his voice and asked: 'Mrs Jones?' Back came a matter of fact reply: 'No, she lives next door'.

Whatever detailed arrangements the doctor makes, they can be great time-savers, speeding up his day. They will not always yield an experience like the above, to lighten his work with laughter.

So much for out of hours' calls. Considerable pressure can also be experienced by the visit requests that come in during working hours. These requests produce various problems, especially when they come during consulting time. Can this discomfort be eased? All doctors deal with these requests in different ways but, in order to raise some of the issues, here is my preferred way of working. The receptionist answers the telephone and asks the patient if he can come to the surgery, offering the carrot that the patient will be seen that morning or that he will be fitted in shortly after arrival. If the caller is not happy to attend, he is put on 'hold' and I am told about the call. If it is convenient I take the call then and there, but otherwise I ask if I can ring back and I do so as soon as the patient I am seeing leaves. I ask what the problem is and listen to the story. I use the same parameters as those already described in the discussion on out of hours' telephone calls: either I say I want to see the patient and ask if he can come in, or I discover I need to visit. If I am clear that the patient could come to surgery I say so, and may also offer to slot him in next after arrival. I am clear that discussions and negotiations can be more thorough if undertaken by a doctor, who of course, only needs to be involved after the receptionist has first sorted things through as far as possible, and even that stage may be more thorough when subsequently the call may be put through to a doctor. If the patient telephoning agrees to come to the surgery, it is easiest if their appointment is tagged onto the end of surgery time, so by telephoning back almost immediately, I give time for the patient to arrive before the surgery ends and I do not then have to hang around waiting for them.

Some doctors do not want the receptionist to disturb them during consultation time. However, my focus is on the whole day's disruption and on the ongoing education of the practice rather than the consultation time alone. I feel my time is finite and worth saving. Saved from waiting or from seeing a patient unnecessarily at their home, my energy is reserved for dealing with other people. For me, the longer-term good outweighs the shorter-term nuisance of interruption to a consultation. Also, the time per consultation can be adjusted to allow for these disturbances if the doctor's day is not so full of house visits. It means the appointment times given to patients in advance may not be so well adhered to, but there is no reason why the doctor should feel he must protect patients from the unpredictability of work with illness.

I am clear that consistent use of this approach educates the population, and steadily the practice settles down. It all needs inter-partner discussion and adjustment, and it needs staff discussion and training, and these adjustments are also reflected in the community. No doubt what I do will change further, but this is how I prefer it now.

Another system we have recently started is in relation to later requests for appointments when some urgency is indicated. We have our pre-booked appointments at ten-minute intervals until a coffee break. We then see patients who say they must be seen that day. They are told they have 'an emergency appointment of five minutes only'. They are then clear that they will have a short appointment and if, for instance, they produce a shopping list of problems, they are told they need to make another appointment for the non-urgent things. After all, in other walks of life appointments are normally made at the convenience of everyone concerned. Under this system the doctor is clear which people consider their problem to be urgent and is in a position to act accordingly, or to point out if the urgent appointment is being abused. The staff find the system easy to work as it is clear, and the patients soon get to know it and respect it.

One doctor I know has arranged that private patients be asked how long they want their appointments to take. He finds patients are quite good at estimating this, so that it saves him time, and in any case they are charged according to time. On the other hand, it can be helpful if only the doctor – and not a receptionist – initiates appointments for longer than the basic ten minutes. The usual ten-minute appointments are in effect a sifting time and for handling those problems that are more quickly sorted. 'I need more time than we have this morning to talk this through, Mr. Smith. Can you come back for thirty minutes tomorrow afternoon, and meanwhile think over what we have already gone over?' Non life-threatening things can best be sorted out when there is no undue pressure of time.

I am sure every group of doctors will have thought through other useful ways of serving people which reduce the stress on themselves and, as a result, in the longer term make for a more effective service. What is clear to me is that it is well worthwhile, both for the population served and for the doctors, that they examine what they aim to do and experiment with how they can move towards their preferred situation.

CHAPTER 5

The Doctor in the Consultation – Man, Machine or God?

Doctors sometimes say half jokingly that they would enjoy medicine far more if it wasn't for their patients, and some go on to further define the situation by adding that if it wasn't for the attitudes of certain patients and sections of society towards them, their lives would be altogether different. Certainly most doctors will observe that a relatively small number of people produce work out of all proportion to their number and medical conditions but, paradoxically, what is at least as important as patient attitudes are three sets of attitudes that are held by doctors. These are: a doctor's self-perception, his beliefs about the role of doctor and his attitudes towards patients. All will have remarkable effects on the doctor/patient relationship and on the way doctors themselves are affected by their work.

It will be convenient for clarity's sake to consider each of these areas separately, but clearly each has considerable bearing on the other and, of course, all meet together in the person of the doctor. This chapter will explore something of the first of these areas, that of the doctor's attitudes to himself, and the other two will be considered in chapters 6 and 12 respectively.

There are many different sorts of people who choose to be doctors and without doubt they will hold many different attitudes, but most want to work with people, want to relate closely and find personal work very satisfying. They see what they do as being for other people. They wish to listen well, to understand and, when medical science cannot cure, to help people adjust to their bodies' limitations. To my mind this is a realistic motivation. It gives place for the individual's humanity and for trust, and has a deeper value than the monetary gain that seems to be the motivation presently encouraged and growing in society. And yet this humanitarian motivation can have an unrealistic ideal added to it.

Within this general attitude of wishing to be of use to people, some doctors feel that, since their work is for the patient, there is no space for themselves in their work. It is as if they find that working for other people means that their own time is not only clearly but exclusively for the patient, and that the doctor is not free to be himself as he searches to function for the patient's good. There seems little concept of there being a whole spectrum of possibilities here, and of there being movement in the doctor/patient relationship. This inflexibility can result in considerable tension. Is there no space for the doctor in the consultation?

Consider first the two extremes of that spectrum. At one end are the doctors who are all in their notes or computers, are centred in tests and medications, all into being clinical, as if they are *all* doctor with little space for themselves as people in their role, and maybe little space for the patient as a person either. They are, no doubt, keeping their distance from illness, defending themselves from their feelings about disease and only able to function with ill patients by erecting such defences. It is unfortunate, however, if their defences spill over so that the doctor is unable to take account of the person in the patient and in himself. At the other end of the spectrum are doctors who are all into listening, into caring and concern for the patient; they are full of sensitivity to the patient as a person, but they too give little space for themselves as people.

Both these groups of people represent extremes in attitude and are probably defences against the doctor's being aware of his own personal sensitivities, vulnerability, distress, and fear of illness and death.

The same attitude is to be found reflected in some partnerships. Partnerships are comprised, of course, of doctors who have selected each other to join in a team and they therefore often hold similar attitudes. One shared attitude can be that if patients are to be properly cared for, the doctors' needs must have little place in the equation.

There will of course be other dynamics within these practices. For instance, there may be the further attitude in one or other member that their own view about patients' needs are clearly right, and this attitude may then be used to belittle any proponent of suggestions for change in the practice organization which would recognize a doctors' personal requirements. The statement: 'Patients need this or that' can be hard to argue with – although of course it is hard to verify too. Often a combination of 'things must *all* be for the good of the patient' and 'I know what patients need' can be used as a tool for control. The controlling doctor's attitude may result in statements like, 'It is ridiculous to suggest such a change in the management of our practice. It would obviously undermine what we are here to do, the whole point of our work. Here we put patients first and we don't want to let our standards slip.' So maintenance of the status quo and the personal defences of that one doctor are hidden behind a banner of 'good patient care'.

An individual doctor who has recently begun to feel there is no space for himself and, as a result, has begun to discuss ways to alter the practice organization to remedy this, may find his previous attitudes strongly held by his partners. There will also be similar controlling and manipulative pressures from outspoken colleagues in the hospital system, as well as patients and politicians who press equivalent opinions. These people's typically outspoken attitudes will serve to reinforce those in the doctor's partners, and yet the spoken pressures from these sources need balancing against the non-pressuring, healthier attitudes that also exist in society, and which are less frequently and more softly spoken, are without manipulative intent and allow the individual freedom to be himself in his work.

Patient care needs to be for its own sake rather than for the maintenance of the doctors' unconscious defences, and to be flexible to the changing circumstances of both doctor and patient. At the same time, all-or-nothing doctors do not get depth of satisfaction from their work as they strive for impossible standards that are inappropriate to both the patient and themselves. It is sad for both parties, as neither patient nor doctor can have a real sense of being able to be there for themselves.

What is the reality of this situation between doctor and patient? They have made a contract; one to be the patient, who comes for time focused on himself and his needs; the other to be the doctor who gives focused time to the patient. In the background lies the fact that a contract can be terminated. Patients often opt out, for instance, by not returning. Doctors, however, are responsible people and their professional concern and stance often means that terminating the contract can feel impossible for them. Yet if the psychological aspect of patient care is under consideration, where of course there is no acute life-threatening physical illness involved, and if, as is usually the case, the doctor is not the only medically qualified person available, terminating the contract may well be the best solution. It would always be a carefully considered step but sometimes it is in the best interests of both parties. For instance, some patients are not only very unpleasant to deal with but can behave very inconsiderately or be repeatedly demeaning and downright offensive. If a doctor can find no way of handling the situation to the patient's benefit, then it would probably be best for another doctor to take the patient on by referral or, if necessary, by the patient being asked to go to another practice. Often it will mean requesting that the patient change practices as the doctors in a group will operate a rota for out of hours' work, so that the particular doctor who is on call may have to attend to any one of his partner's patients. This is not to punish the patient nor is it a situation of failure, but of good sense. But be that as it may, what is important here is that the doctor needs to hold fast to the notion that he does have the choice and freedom to accept or reject the patient who is now in front of him for care. There is no compulsion for the doctor to take care of an individual patient, and therefore there is no place for the doctor to feel trapped. In itself, this realization has a freeing effect of value to both parties and to the work done.

Every doctor, despite good and flexible organization, will have times when he is overstretched. Years ago I was called to a road accident during an evening surgery. I found myself by the roadside, intubating an unconscious, blue patient and setting up an intravenous drip. The injuries were grisly and distressing. The procedures in the cold and in dwindling evening light were difficult and exacting, and necessitated sitting on the wet ground. The whole process was made emotionally fraught because the passenger was crying, both because of her pain and out of anxiety for her husband. None of the people present on the rough grass of that country roadside could have been unmoved by the experience: all were shocked, distressed and emotionally drained.

Afterwards I returned to the surgery to find a group of patients dutifully awaiting my return. I put my head around the waiting room door to be greeted with a cheerful chorus, 'Don't worry doctor, we're all waiting for you.' At that moment I knew I had had enough, and for the first time found myself saying, 'I'm sorry, but I just can't see you tonight. I need to see Mr Smith urgently, but otherwise please arrange other appointments unless you feel it's urgent to see me.' That was a breakthrough for me: a breakthrough to a realisation that patients need the full person of the doctor and that I wasn't a god. If the doctor is only half there, he is of little use. I am clear there are times when, for their own sakes as much as for the doctor's, patients may need to be asked to return another time if their condition is not absolutely urgent. The reality is that the doctor's job includes the unexpected and urgent, and these stresses do not need to be kept hidden from patients, nor patients to be protected from the reality of the doctor's life.

A somewhat complex example will develop the theme. Some years back, when I was first experimenting with videoing my own and my trainee's consultations, it became clear that my Indian doctor trainee, in the consultation which she had brought to show and discuss, had shut herself off from the patient. It was as if she suddenly switched off and became unavailable. In response to my questions she said that she was imagining herself on a hillside on an Indian evening, feeling the cool breeze through her hair and over the nape of her neck, a delicious place in her imaginings.

It transpired that the morning surgery she had videoed had been a heavy one and she had been overstretched even before the consultation we were now viewing had taken place. She then found herself confronted by the rantings of a highly judgemental and controlling patient. She had found this to be the last straw and needed to protect herself. She could not cope with the way she was being treated by the patient, and she shut off.

And why not? She could learn from the situation, just as the patient could also learn from it. I hope she learned to regulate her surgery length to what she could cope with; to plan appropriate breaks in her work; and to feel free to walk into another room and have an unplanned cup of coffee when she needed a break. If the day is proving too heavy, the doctor becomes defensive and of little use to the patient.

Returning to the discussion with the trainee over her videoed consultation; there is a process of reflection that occurs when a doctor discusses his work with a colleague. It is as if he models for his colleague to experience in their discussion the dilemma the patient first brought to the consultation, as if the feelings engendered in the room when the doctor was seeing the patient are again brought to life as the consultation is discussed between the doctor and his colleague. The interaction between the two doctors contains the same elements as the initial interaction in the consultation between the patient and doctor. In psychotherapy terminology this is called the 'reflection process' or 'parallel process', and it is a fundamental tool in casework supervision (Mattinson, 1975). Working with it makes the casework discussion alive, and enables a doctor's work in supervision to move to a more effective level and deeper understanding.

This reflection process can usefully be applied to the discussion with the trainee doctor about her videoed consultation. She had found herself switching off from the patient, and as we discussed the consultation I found that I wanted to switch off from our discussion too. When the trainee spoke of imagining herself on an Indian hillside, it transported me in my turn to an occasion when I had stood one evening on a hill overlooking the bay on which Bombay stands. The lights of the city were winking and reflected in the calm sea, and a gentle evening breeze cooled my over-heated face after what had been a two day, nightmare journey of travel disasters, heat, noise and weariness. Reviewing the consultation I, too, became aware of a need to escape. Both of us could consider it idle day-dreaming, but if this was in fact the reflection process at work, then it would have been the patient's own experiences and leftover feelings of needing to get away that first stimulated the need in her doctor to escape into fantasies of cool, breathable air, and which we now felt and suffered in the supervision discussion. We could speculate that in this patient's past she would repeatedly have endured suffocating experiences, perhaps of coercion, that now lived on in her, so that she longed to escape from unpleasant restriction to pleasant havens with breathable, life-sustaining air. Now if the reflection process is valid, it can be seen that it is one that provides a most powerful and vivid communication, and it means that the doctor's feelings, fantasies and apparent attention-slips are all to be monitored because they can have a considerable impact on his understanding of the patient.

As has been said, a succession of young doctors have puzzled over how they can be wholly themselves in consultations set up for the patient. Roger Neighbour, in his book, *The Inner Consultation* (1987), seems to me to be struggling with this, though not at this depth. He advocates exercises to coerce the mind to stay fixed on the patient. It feels like 'Do a hundred lines for letting your mind wander.' If this is so, it seems to be advocating control of a large part of the doctor's person. Clearly it is only one option and one that limits the doctor so that he loses out on the pleasure of two human beings trying to interact fully with each other, using every part of themselves, including memories, fantasy and feelings. Rather than control, could not the doctor aim to be free to explore and use whatever he finds going on in him? Is there not a full place for the person of the doctor in the consultation?

There is another facet to this. Patrick Casement has written and explored his idea of an 'internal supervisor' (1985). In psychotherapy the mulling over of one's work is held to be essential and is done on a regular basis with an experienced colleague, commonly called a supervisor. Casement explores the concept of having an internal conversation while the consultation is in progress to, as it were, discuss with an 'internal supervisor' what is happening and the options available. He sees this internal supervisor as being there not to judge or be obeyed, but to engage with in a process of internally putting into words the thoughts, feelings and images experienced in relation to what the patient says and does. In this internal discussion the doctor looks for his own feeling reactions and then formulates possible verbal responses to the patient. It enables him to consider the most likely effect on the patient of his proposed verbal interventions, and to choose the response that he judges most likely to be accepted and effective.

A similar internal search and mulling over of options can be usefully employed by doctors. For example, the trainee doctor with her consultation video-recording referred to above, could consciously have used this technique. The patient was in essence haranguing the doctor about a series of consultations that had taken place over a number of years and with a number of colleagues. She had never returned to the same doctor twice if she could help it and her 'disease' had never improved. She clearly implied that she felt the various doctors had not done their job. She had a whole list of troubles that seemed to include every organ in her body. The verbal flow of complaint about her body went on and on, and she always sounded displeased and critical of her body, her doctors and of everything around her. She experienced life as if it were out of step and certainly did not even remotely entertain the thought that she was herself out of step with the world. There was an implied threat that this new doctor was quickly, if not already, to be added to the list of those who had failed her.

What were the doctor's options? Certainly she could pull her prescription pad towards her and have the patient leave with the promise of help from some new medication. In the short term that would certainly shorten and relieve the doctor's discomfort. Alternatively the doctor could choose one problem and refer the patient to a specialist. This would 'prove' interest without having to prolong the consultation. Again, the doctor could set up some tests partly, no doubt, because they might be relevant and partly again to 'prove' interest. Or the doctor could reflect on the whole patient, her physical pains, her pressurising distress and the distressed feelings the patient produced in her, and opt to try and deal with the total person. She could draw the patient into making a list of her troubles, offering to deal with them in the order of the patient's priority and, over a succession of consultations, gently challenge the patient to reconsider her attitudes. I am sure there are other options, but the point I want to make here is that we are now functioning as if we are having a discussion with an internal supervisor, mulling over the causes of what is happening and the possible options for the doctor. Similarly the trainee doctor whose case this was might have asked herself: 'What is needed by this patient and what approach might reach across her defensive wall? What first step might I make towards a realistic long-term goal which might be acceptable to this patient?' With time a doctor can gain confidence in the validity of the link between the doctor's inner world and the patient's, and so progressively dare to voice the unspoken.

I will surmise that the doctor is willing to take on the challenge of the consultation, chooses to take a long view of the problem and, as a result of the understandings gained through the reflection process, sees the patient's probable past experience of suffering. She might then put out one or two feelers to test the patient's motivation. If she did this she might find that the patient is not totally averse to dictating a clear list of symptoms and to returning to work on them at successive consultations. The doctor is encouraged to try putting some thoughts forward about the patient's feeling state, and floats the idea that perhaps she is quite distressed that so much seems to be going wrong with her. 'Yes,' says the patient 'I am annoyed you don't seem to be doing very much to help me.' At least the patient is owning a feeling, although she is blaming the doctor for it. The doctor makes a mental note to take this a step further next time, and finishes by asking the patient to return on a specific day in a week's time. The patient leaves with the inkling that this doctor is taking her seriously, but she must be prepared to return and give the process time and a chance. If the patient returns, then, over several interviews, it is possible that the feelings so disruptive to the patient's life may be put into words, given their due value and owned as her own. Possibly a process will have begun that, with time, may enable the various strands of this person to come together. To my mind it would be a worthwhile aim to have this patient take a telephone number so as to contact a psychotherapist, but I am sure this would not be acceptable for a long time to come.

This is an example of the doctor using all his internal processes – his sensitivity of feeling, his inner responses and his thought processes – to enable appropriate selection and action to be taken by one small step at a time in an experimental trial, while being prepared to withdraw and try another approach as necessary. It is a difficult task, but it represents a mode of operation that involves the doctor fully. All parts of his nature are integrated. The patient may tell the doctor what she thinks, feels and does, and the doctor uses what is said but also brings himself into the consultation through using his feeling response to all the patient brings – or fails to bring – into the room. Fantasies and feelings make the understanding deeper and more complete. The doctor's options and choices are internally monitored for their effectiveness.

It follows from this that a doctor can usefully be open to experience his feelings during the consultation. He needs to clarify which are his own and which come from the patient's past. He needs to give feeling and fantasy the importance of being relevant in communication. He does not need to control or remove them, and certainly they are not to be censured or restricted. It is important for both patient and doctor that he remains a full, unrestricted human being and thereby shows the patient how it is possible for her also to remain herself. He models that it is possible and acceptable for the doctor to break out of succumbing to another's manipulation, and that therefore it is acceptable for the patient to do the same and react quite differently from the way she has repeatedly done in the past.

Every part of the doctor is legitimately used. He enters fully into the detective puzzle which the patient has brought. There is constant movement in the interaction. Doctor boredom and any sense of failure disappear as realistic goals for the individual consultation are made and often attained. The doctor can be himself, and of course his self-perception will remarkably affect his work.

With this model of working there is place for the full person of the doctor. At the same time it is apparent that the full person will include experiencing painful, distressing and very uncomfortable feelings, but if he can let himself experience these, he will also be able to use them.

I hope this chapter has demonstrated that, just as a doctor's work makes a great impact on his life, so his self-perception will remarkably affect his work.

CHAPTER 6

The Doctor's Role

The last chapter sought to demonstrate that the way in which doctors think of themselves will affect their work, and this chapter follows on from that by exploring a family doctor's view of his role in the psychological areas of his work. Towards the end of the book, a doctor's attitudes to patients will also be considered, but while all these attitudinal aspects have an interrelating effect, this chapter's focus is on the doctor's role.

What a doctor does in the psychological area of his work depends on what he makes of his role. He cannot choose whether or not to be involved in this area: he is. Yet in the end there is no fixed, right, invariable and definitive description, and when an attempt is made to describe his role, it cannot possibly do justice to what the doctor is doing in the next room. It would only be an exposition of one person's attitudes as he seeks to grapple with those of each individual patient.

However, if each doctor attempts to define his role then it is at least conceivable that it would relieve him from concerns that lie outside it. Having said that, the family doctor's role with regard to the patient's psyche can be immensely variable if the doctor adjusts to the wide variety of human problems brought to him. The greater his experience and the more flexible he is, the wider his role can become.

This will sound daunting if it is taken to mean that a doctor's work will have no boundaries and require endless time and energy. And this would probably be so except that as he gains experience he is more able to discern the root cause of the problems brought to him. He is therefore able to select an effective focus more accurately and to choose the skills that he now can judge to be most likely to be useful. Therefore, the more flexible the doctor can be with his methods of work, and the more he is able to work at a deeper level when it is appropriate, the less time and energy he will use up in the longer term. He uses time to greater effect.

To define the doctor's job widely, therefore, is to describe the breadth and interest of his work spread over many patients. His role will include choosing the most appropriate focus and method, and he must judge when it would be reasonable, both to himself and to the patient, for him to undertake the treatment or, alternatively, to

59

choose another skilled person who can help. He will need to be mature enough to accept that he cannot be all things to all people and therefore be at ease with referring patients to a well trained and experienced psychotherapist or counsellor just as, in other circumstances, he would to a medical specialist or surgeon. The more accurately the doctor fulfils the role appropriate to a patient's situation, or draws in someone else who can, the sooner that patient will leave satisfied and not need to return. With these beliefs in mind, I would like to explore the doctor's role.

Doctors, along with other helping professions, are largely a self-selected group by virtue of a common wish to be of service to those who are ill. Further, they are then trained for action on behalf of the patient. It is important, for example, that a doctor lets out the pus, or treats heart failure; that he treat the patient's physical ills. It is also important that he work to support patients too debilitated to cope with their social problems: when, for instance, people are not able to help themselves he needs to step in and support their application for urgent housing, or to admit the psychotic to a place of safety. The young, the elderly and the mentally disabled may rightly need his active participation. Where, though, does his activity lie in the area of the psyche? Other than in physical medicine, is it helpful for a doctor to be busy on the patient's behalf and, if so, in what way? Can a doctor's own need to be active get in the way?

When I first came into family practice I really had no experience of psychiatry at all, and I remember the first patient I referred to a psychiatrist. I wondered what she would say to my suggestion of a referral and was surprised that she did not take offence. Clearly for me at that time, being distraught to the point of feeling in some way mad was not something I saw as a feeling we all have within us somewhere, but rather as something which it would be better not to allow and certainly not be admitted. Anyway, she was happy to go to see a psychiatrist and I arranged that I would see her again after her appointment. When she came back I remember asking with considerable interest how she had got on. 'Oh fine, I am to go again.' 'Yes, but what happened?' 'Oh it was quite interesting really. He let me talk and after a time I realised the poor man had gone to sleep with his head on his hands. Anyway I carried on till I had told him all I wanted and then I coughed and shuffled my feet, and he woke up and said that he thought we should leave it there for now and I should see him again in two weeks. The strange thing is, I feel very much better for it.'

I think this was the first inkling I had that in matters of the mind the doctor does not actively have to do something. What is it, then, that he does, or is, for the patient?

If the doctor is active – even only by talking – then the patient is passively listening. Yet the problem is the patient's. Doctors must feel free not to attempt to answer questions but rather to pose them for the patient. The need is for the problems to be owned by the patient, for the problems to be explored and understood by them, and then dealt with by the person whose problem it is. The patient has come to think it through by talking. In the end nothing else can be satisfactory. People are stuck in problems because they are in a phase of not dealing with them. That is their more fundamental difficulty, more basic than the outside problem they ostensibly bring to their doctor. They bring a problem they are stuck with to demonstrate that they cannot work through their problems. Sort one for them and they become stuck with the next. Seen this way the doctor's task shifts from solving the immediate problem for the patient to supporting the patient as he discovers why he is not doing his own problem solving. The doctor's task shifts to facilitating the inner processes and to the definition of the deeper problem. For this it is necessary to sample the feelings involved and get them out into the open. They clarify the patient's inner needs. Then the patient can be left to work through his options and, in his own time, take any action that may be appropriate.

Some patients may then go away and sort themselves out on their own. Others, however, cannot do this. It is as if they have not yet developed the ability to stand back from their lives and take time to decide on management issues that enable them to take a desired new direction. It is as if these people need their attention holding by the doctor in just such a stand-back-and-make-decisions mode of operation. The doctor holds a space for them to function in this new way. He needs to trust in the human processes of change and must allow the patient to make his own timorous step from, for instance, the second rung of some ladder of change, to the third. He needs to be content with this, even though he knows there are many more rungs to the ladder. The patient can climb only one step at a time and it is the patient who must take the steps in this new process. It is the patient who must first trust each rung of the ladder before he can reasonably try it with his weight. For this he may need the doctor there, just to be there with him and taking pleasure in his new skills.

I wonder if the reader has had the experience of talking about something for the first time and finding that as you talked you were surprised at what came out, as if it was not known to you until it was said. It is as if you discover what goes on in you through putting it into words. I understand this is a fairly universal human experience. That being so, what deprivation an individual suffers if he does not have, or allow himself, someone with whom to discuss and talk. I suspect, therefore, that something of what a doctor does is just to be with the patient, daring to stay while they speak of their hopes and fears, their worries, their unmentionable or unbearable secrets, their pain and distress; to stay while they are discovering through their talking. If the doctor gives these things importance, then perhaps the patient can too. If the doctor can bear to hear of the patient's distresses, the patient may believe he can too. If the doctor can remain there, the patient's thoughts, and even they themselves, become acceptable or worthy of consideration. If the doctor gives time to listening, the patient can discover himself as he puts things into words for the first time, and if the doctor does not immediately prescribe antidepressants, then the message is that their depression, their feeling of the moment, is all right, is part of life, does not need control but just room to be – for as long as it takes. Action by the doctor is not required, but rather recognition of feeling as being part of the human condition.

When feelings are recognized people can take them into account in their decision-making. They can recognize that part of themselves, value themselves, use themselves and live more fully. Part of the doctor's activity is the recognition of the full person and a taking of that whole person seriously. It will include pointing out significant silent places, 'You have not told me of your father's part in this', or pointing out significant silence in feeling areas, 'You haven't told me what effect this had on you. How did it make you feel?' People respond internally to every event in life. These feelings are all part of the experience. People have not told the whole of the story until the internal impact is also uncovered. The reason for recounting an episode becomes clear as the personal involvement and the feelings engendered are clarified.

Recognition and verbal handling of feelings by the doctor also enables work on projected feelings, as is indicated in later chapters. Patients can be encouraged to acknowledge and carry their own feelings as a result, and so become more fully themselves and more free to act appropriately.

Once a patient who is unused to acknowledging his feelings samples this focus on his inner self, he will often have a sense of self-discovery and liberation that may result in a wish to move on to his own psychotherapy or analysis.

Doctors will surely come up against patients' perceptions of what they believe and see as the doctor's role which differ from their own. I remember going to see a woman in her late twenties who had just had her first baby. She had rung me because the baby was not feeding properly and was crying a great deal. They had fairly recently moved to the village and as I entered the garden I noted the beautiful rich texture of the local stone of the house and the snug thatched roof. The well-oiled gate had recently been made from rustic oak, and the flag path was now beautifully laid and edged with brick. Around the door was a climbing rose and, yes, it was a thornless variety. As I talked to her it became apparent that her new baby was expected to adapt, and be tidy and bloom peacefully like the house. I sat down with her and over a cup of tea slowly painted a picture of her adapting to the baby's needs. Slowly she became quieter, and then there burst out of her with considerable anger: 'You are a doctor. You are supposed to make me feel better.'

The doctor's role will conflict with the patient's wishes often enough. What the patient wants and what they need to face may not be the same. A doctor will need, on the one hand, a flexible sensitivity to adjust to each patient where they are today (with an ability to get alongside them and make good rapport), and on the other he will need a firmness to challenge the same patient to make similar adjustments to their perceptions and expectations in their longer-term life. For this the doctor will need a knowledge and understanding of human personality development so that his role can be to clarify the patients' realities and make it more difficult for them to duck or delay facing the challenges life presents. The journalist Hugo Young refers, in an article in *The Guardian* (22 December 1994) written on quite a different subject, to 'the bedside smirk of reassurance'. What patients require is the encouragement and wherewithal to face reality.

It seems to me that one of the adjustments I have made down the years is a quite major one of progressively attributing more importance to the self-imposed cause of many physical illnesses. I see this as part of keeping patients responsible for as much of their lives as possible. The more responsibility a person takes for his life, the more able he is to give it shape. It becomes more and more *his* life. He can figuratively take it by the scruff of the neck and walk it down his chosen road.

Certainly there are those who would prefer not to feel responsible. After all, taking responsibility requires effort and can be frightening; it involves letting go of dependency; it calls for action that some find difficult to take for fear of being seen to be responsible for the consequences; it demands they look at their anxieties to find the inner forces that sway them, and to work to free themselves to become full persons. It demands much, but that is better than hanging about, blowing with the wind, complaining whenever they end up somewhere they do not like to be.

They complain at authority figures (who they perceive as being responsible), and envy the recognition that is given to people who are active and who make the most of their situation.

One way that people may limit themselves is to blame life for their state. A wiry thirty-five-year-old businessman came in to see his doctor with quick steps and darting eyes. He looked at his watch as if to emphasize that he had been kept waiting some ten minutes and told his doctor he would not keep him long. He was not sleeping, he said, and wanted some sleeping tablets for when he was staying in hotels on his business trips.

The doctor talked over a typical night and it became apparent that the man's sleeping pattern was interrupted all the time and not just when he was in a strange beds. He would get up and smoke and, as he sat there talking in the consultation, his nervous tension was apparent as he fidgeted with his watch and picked at the skin folds of his nails. No, he did not plan on taking a holiday. He had not had one for three years. He lived in a pub which his wife ran, and he helped with the pub work whenever he was at home. The time came for the doctor to give his feedback to the patient and he remarked on how stressful it was to moonlight and do two jobs, especially when one of them was actually a business run in his own home. Oh, he had no problem with that; they were used to it. He and his wife had come to live in their present pub from a similar sort of situation.

It was hard work for the doctor to get this A1, fast-lane type personality to see that his behaviour was not in his body's best interests, even if, in the short term, his bank balance improved with it; nor that he could not really expect to be able to keep up such a pace, that he was running down his batteries, and that those batteries were not as able to hold their charge as well as they had done even a few years previously. It turned out that his contempt for his physical needs also extended to excess alcohol consumption, smoking, short nights and taking meals on the run, all of which resulted in frequent, prolonged indigestion and chestiness. This man's physical symptoms arose out of his attitude to himself. It was as if he denied that he was more than a work-horse and denied both his need, and the challenge, of deeper, sustaining relationships. He blamed his body; it was not his fault.

In dealing with him it was as if his doctor had first to see, and then to hold, the total person the patient was; hold onto those parts and the needs he denied, keeping them present in the room for him to slowly recognize until he could acknowledge them and allow them a place in his life (Joseph, 1985). Here the concept of the unconscious is important (Freud, 1915). It is as if the patient had no knowledge of his need and yet, with time, people do discover needs and forces that were there all along.

In this instance the doctor's role was to recognize what was missing, to see that the man's various stresses were a deeper cause for his disturbed nights than his travelling. Life's developmental journey includes the need for the freedom to be a full person. This man seemed unconscious of this. The more he discovered parts of himself made conscious through being put into words, the more he could throw off his symptoms along the way.

A doctor's role may at times demand the ability to see beyond and beneath what the patient presents as his problem, to know not only the norms for the body but also the norms in human personality development terms; to treat the symptom and relieve physical discomfort but then pass on to concentrate on deeper needs. Some investigations may then become unnecessary.

Patients with A1-type personalities who blame everything else but themselves, can be hard work. The doctor must catch hold of them as they race past, press them to sit awhile, invite them to take a deep breath and sample the morning air, to notice that the sun is shining and a thrush singing. Do they notice that their food has taste; that their partner is smiling with them, not laughing at them; indeed, do they know that sex can be more than the relief of tension in hurried orgasm? It is as if life consists of doing, with no place for quiet reflection and letting life sink in, no place for it to be an experience full of feeling and contemplation. The three parts of a man – his thinking, feeling and doing – have not yet been discovered by them so that they, as persons, are not whole. They exist to do, hardly allowing their thinking part, and denying their feelings.

There are, of course, opposite types of patient. I remember a man who had had Crohn's disease since his teens. Crohn's can be looked on as characterized by successive, over-developed, knotted muscle masses that obstruct the flow of food, and which have formed in gut muscle that has been too long tensed and uptight. The diagnosis was made when he had an operation for suspected acute appendicitis, after which he developed various complications including a bursting of the gut to the surface of the skin with chronic discharge. For some time he had been well enough in himself, but he repeatedly experienced painful partial obstruction requiring hospital admission. One day, as I gave him time to reflect on life, he said, 'You know doctor, I think this is a lot to do with tension. I'm quite all right unless I do something that worries me or something happens in the family that gets me up tight. When that happens I've come to recognize that my pain will start with this partial obstruction and, unless I can calm down, I'm in hospital again.'

Here is a patient who has now become conscious of his feelings, thinks about himself and then takes action that can relax his gut. He has become quite the opposite to the A1 personality described previously.

But let's speculate, for it cannot be much more than that. Could it be that as a boy, this patient was so uptight that the nervous gut contractions that produce the diarrhoea that so many people know about when they are anxious, became a literal knotting-up of his gut that was so continuous that it resulted in the permanent changes of Crohn's disease? It would then be as if this patient's body was insisting on his recognition of tension and distress, demanding he be aware of himself.

I remember being fascinated by the following. I am not sure now where I read it but the writer was exploring possible physical illnesses that might develop because of patient attitudes. He postulated as follows. When a baby is being fed, its stomach will secrete acid so as to do its job in digesting its food. While the baby is fed, mother is also lovingly handling it, cuddling and perhaps talking soothingly, giving the infant considerable loving care and attention. Could it not be, he suggested, that for some people in later life, the need for loving care might trigger acid secretion quite irrespective of the need for food or the proximity of meal times? Could it not be as if, Pavlovian style, the stomach has learnt to respond to the human need for attention rather than to the smell or ingestion of food?

If this is a factor in a particular patient, then the doctor's usual physical treatments for stomach acidity are clearly symptomatic in character. If the patient can recognize his needs and take up a lifestyle that enables him to ask for – and receive – love and care, then he may be able to re-train his stomach to respond to food needs only. The patient would then be both understanding himself and taking up responsibility for his well-being.

Yet a further example is that of rheumatoid arthritis seen as developing in people with difficulty in expressing their anger. It could well be that the tenseness of muscles in these people – tense with much unexpressed or unconscious anger – would so constantly pressurise their joints that the joint lining eventually reacts with an inflammatory response which, if prolonged, is followed by the permanent rheumatoid joint changes. Certainly I am struck by how usual it is for people with this diagnosis to feel trapped in their lives and to have a smouldering sense of dissatisfaction that is often hidden behind a smiling, passive exterior.

It may be that the reader will wish to explore this effect of the dynamics of human relationships further. Dr Kenneth Sanders, general practitioner and psychoanalyst, in his book, *A Matter of Interest* (1986), and June Mainprice in her book, *Marital Interaction and Some Illnesses in Children* (1974) (to mention two of many books), provide some further examples of the psychological causes of physical symptoms, and Doctors Norman Cameron and Joseph Rychlak give a comprehensive view of developmental pitfalls of the personality in their book, *Personality Development and Psychopathology* (1985).

Belief that physical illnesses are frequently a symptom of internal conflicts alters the role of the doctor. It then becomes relevant to draw a patient into exploring insights into their psyche and to invite reflection on their own responsibility for their symptoms. The patient will need time to consider a change in their attitude and so effect change in their behaviour. Their changed understanding may bring relief from their physical symptoms, but also can bring relief to their distressed psyche too.

It should not be surprising if patients bring their difficulties to the doctor in various ways. They may bring their concern verbally and, when they do, they have clearly given permission to talk about that concern, so that the doctor will usually feel at ease in addressing it. However, many patients cannot talk about themselves. They have not learnt to express their inner problems. They may come because, perhaps unconsciously, they expect to have some inner door oiled and the key found. The doctor's role may then be to put his sense of their problem into words so that it can be firmed up and verbally handled and worked on.

Some who cannot speak may bring their problems as pains and symptoms (Balint, M., 1957). Perhaps, as a small child, their concerns were not recognized but, when translated into tummy pain, at least they were kept home from school and a parent put himself out, just a little, to bring medicine or a drink to their bed.

Whatever the way a patient presents his problem to the doctor, its root cause needs search and discussion and, above all, it needs putting into words. For instance, the patient with indigestion needs his stomach examining but also his anxiety both accepting and pin-pointing. 'Your stomach is all right – I have looked into that – but tell me about yourself. Oh, so your wife is busy with her business and has no time for you and the family. She is getting more and more involved in her work. You do not feel she hears your concern of the family's need for more of her time at home and less of the tired, preoccupied her. What you have said to her has not had any effect. It is the same as when your words failed you as a child. But now of course, as an adult, you can be more forceful, you can more successfully strive to find the words to persuade and put your point of view.' You, the doctor, can suggest the mature way of interacting to replace the ineffective, tongue-tied childhood way.

This is clearly over-simplified and contracted, but the doctor's role is to make a diagnosis, whether physical, psychological or both, and put them on the table. Then the patient can decide what he does about it.

The conversation with a hypochondriac might well go as follows: 'You are very anxious about something: if not about one possible illness then another. It is not physical illness that is your problem, but your excess anxiety. You may need to come again to talk this through, or I could give you the telephone number of a psychotherapist.' The patient will need time to think about this and come again, but they know what the diagnosis is and what they can do to begin to sort it through. Also, of course, the doctor knows that in future, each time he uncovers pathological behaviour, he can refer back to this conversation. 'I wonder if you have thought more about your own psychotherapy.' It removes from the doctor the feeling of responsibility that *he* must do something or that *he* has not sorted something out and that *he* has failed in some way. By keeping the patient responsible for his or her own health, the doctor is not locked into a stagnant relationship, a game of 'pass the responsibility' that gets nowhere fast.

Other patients who cannot speak about themselves may, in their desperation, enact their problem. Their behaviour in the consulting room, if the doctor gets them to focus on it, enables their problems to be put into verbal focus, bringing them self-understanding, maybe, for the first time. For instance, there are the severely controlling patients who dehumanise the doctor and leave him no space to be himself. They can be really infuriating, but with the above hypothesis, it is legitimate ground for discussion. If the patient brings severe control into the consulting room, then, odds on, he is also doing it at home and at work and, as a result, is having a real problem relating closely to people who all back away and clear off, out of his prison. He perhaps knows no other way to relate. In that case he will be confused and lonely. His life is in stalemate. One way or another, his core difficulty in relating needs to be put into words and then perhaps he can begin to discuss it in his family and, as a result, find faith both in himself and humanity. Talking about it relieves his isolation, enables the development of mutual understanding and respect and allows him, as well as those around him, to recognize internal struggles and to develop as persons in their own way.

A further example of a patient bringing his problem as behaviour rather than in words is that of a man who is totally inflexible with the doctor. He may find talking over his difficulty in allowing adaptation very helpful. For the first time he may then begin to accept and understand his wife's frustration with him when he retired and began spending his days at home. He moves nearer to considering those evening classes his neighbour goes to and rediscovering a variety of his old interests to take up once more. Until his inflexibility is recognized by his doctor and brought to his conscious attention, the patient cannot focus on the problem.

There are so many patient behaviours brought as demonstrations to the consulting room. They can usefully be looked at as being brought by the patient for the doctor's observation and help. If the doctor voices what he sees, it will sometimes be received with interest and responded to by the patient with active work, and, sometimes, as with all the doctor's interventions, they will be ignored. Either way, nothing is lost, but a lot may be gained. It demands that the doctor develop an ability to handle different patients in different ways. I don't see this as extra work, but rather as working at a different level, and in different ways, with the variety of problems that different patients bring. The doctor's worthwhile aim is to be free to use one approach with one patient, and another with a different patient; to do nothing with this patient here this time (perhaps because of his own lack of time); and with yet another, to refer as appropriate to a psychotherapist, behavioural therapist or counsellor.

In general the qualifications and functions of counsellors and psychotherapists are often confusing and perhaps they are particularly so to those used to a medical model of treatment. It has been noted elsewhere that doctors frequently have a distrust or uncertainty about referral to professionals in other disciplines who are not qualified doctors and yet, of course, it is the doctor's role to refer people to wherever they can receive the most appropriate and effective help. Appendix 2 gives the addresses of tried and tested national training organizations that doctors can turn to for assistance in assessing more local services.

As a further aside, it is worth recording that it is my experience that, out of some 2,000 patients, to my knowledge twenty or more would be undertaking psychotherapy or counselling at any one time. These people represent those with difficulties who are willing and able to make adjustments with another's help. Once they have made the decision to seek assistance, they then seldom need to attend their doctor except for physical problems.

However, when a patient is not ready to change, at subsequent visits to his family doctor his ongoing, depressed ramblings can be cut short: 'You really do need to ring that psychotherapist you know. What is stopping you?' Holding life's challenges in front of patients keeps them empowered and responsible for as much of their lives as possible. Gone are the repeated consultations with the two locked in confusion by their matching pairs of needs or projections. Gone is the doctor's endless struggle with a sense of his own and the patient's stagnation. Gone are the ongoing heavy feelings in the doctor as if he were in a mire, each step made only by lifting the weight of his mud-coated foot, sucked down by resistant clinging clay.

Clearly this is not a comprehensive picture of the doctor's psychological role. Because of the breadth of the work that would be very difficult. Clearly, too, this is to give some vision that may only be realistic with one patient here and another there, but vision is like the yeast that leavens.

And what I have described is still too much for the doctor to do, too active for the patient's good. Rather, the doctor needs to hold the attitude within himself that each individual is responsible for himself. That is enough.

CHAPTER 7

Using and Being Used by People (Projection)

It is time now to turn to some more immediately practical material that can be applied to work to make it less stressful and more satisfying. This chapter sets a theoretical background for understanding a major part of the stress that comes through working with people; an understanding that can improve the quality of the work undertaken and deepen the satisfaction it brings, as well as reduce the worker's stress. It outlines a theory which subsequent chapters will develop and apply.

Doctors spend a disproportionate amount of time with people with disturbed feelings. There are, for instance, those who are greatly distressed, those who are deeply depressed and those who are having to face unpleasant aspects of their bodies' ageing processes. Frequently these people will at least temporarily turn to their doctor to share their unpleasant feelings and often will unconsciously leave him to carry them on their behalf. Such a process may leave the doctor holding the patient's burden for a considerable length of time, and considering that this experience may be repeated by one patient after another, it can be the source of considerable doctor discomfort.

A business woman came to her doctor. She did not often come but when she did, she proved to be an uncomfortable person to be with. For instance, her doctor had always found her to be suspicious and she was especially questioning of everything he said. Since the doctor's carefully considered style was to give people the information from which to make up their own minds about what course of action they wished to take, her suspicion suggested a considerable distrust. The doctor always found himself making extra effort to give her all the information he could in an attempt to prevent a sense in himself that he was not adequate.

One morning she said she wanted a private referral for a hysterectomy: just that. The doctor had no record of any problems suggesting a hysterectomy might be needed, and the only possible relevant fact he knew was that she was in her mid-forties. He had nothing with which to build up an adequate picture of her difficulties to enable him to advise a suitable referral. He therefore asked if

71

she could tell him what lay behind her request, and was firmly told she just wanted him to refer her to the specialist. It rapidly became clear that, in effect, this was an order. He was not being allowed to be a person in his own right; it was as if he was regarded as a human word-processor, necessary only for mechanically printing a letter – and rather irritating at that.

The doctor could have referred her indiscriminately to any consultant, perhaps with some comment to the specialist that he did not know anything about why she wanted to be seen. This would have been less work for him, but he would also have been forced to act in a way that did not suit or please him. He was already loaded with a sense of dismay at her controlling behaviour, and with feelings that resulted from his being used and manipulated. He could not feel good about himself in this situation and decided to inform her of his predicament. He told her he did not know what sort of special area of interest the specialist would need in order to give her the focused care her condition required. It was probable that some prior investigations might help in deciding which particular specialist would be appropriate. It was the job of her family doctor to investigate to a point where an intelligent choice of specialist was possible, and so on. She resisted, but he stuck to his role and slowly, very slowly, she allowed him to be a doctor and more of a person. At the end of the interview they agreed on a referral. She quickly got her hysterectomy, though for doubtful reasons.

Doctors have frequently told me how de-personalizing and unpleasant they find interviews with people like this. Some have said that they can sour the rest of the day for them. Certainly this doctor put energy and time into the consultation but in the end he felt he had done as well as he could by the patient, and that he had maintained himself so that he was not left loaded with too much unpleasant feeling.

I would like to examine what was happening here and apply a theory that may help with understanding the interaction – and understanding is necessary if doctors are to help themselves to keep free from being used in uncomfortable and therefore stressful ways, and if they are to be of maximum use to patients.

This patient was exerting pressure on her doctor to write a letter as if dictated by her. She expected him to respond to an order without thinking and with little feeling response. It was dehumanizing. I think, too, she was using him to deposit various feelings which she unconsciously (Freud, 1915) could not cope with. For instance, he found himself feeling anxious because he could not see himself happily writing the letter she requested to a consultant colleague without first doing the sorting that forms a necessary part of the family doctor's work. In this there was his own anxiety in relation to the possible serious nature of whatever illness she might have, as well as to what the consultant might think about his work. But he also felt an anxiety which had quite a different feel to it and that was over and above his own. He realised he did not know what was going on in this woman's abdomen and so he felt baffled. Normally he would ask questions and develop an ability to hypothesize. His bafflement and anxiety would ease as he examined and investigated, but this patient would not allow this. It was as if she was pushing over to him her anxiety and bafflement at not knowing. The doctor worked hard to try and develop a satisfactory outcome. Nevertheless he had a sense of being dissatisfied with his work and had a feeling that the patient was not pleased with it either. He therefore speculated that she also offloaded onto him her feeling of dissatisfaction with herself and her body. He had felt annoyed, uncomfortable, used and manipulated; so these feelings, too, may have been ones she could not bear to carry for herself. There was, therefore, a whole load of quite unpleasant feelings that the doctor held and which were not fully relevant to himself, and were disquieting and stress producing.

This process of unloading unwanted feelings onto another person has been given the name of 'projection' (Klein, 1952). It is an unconscious process by the projector, and usually for the person receiving the projection, too. It is a useful concept for doctors. An understanding of it can be used to the patient's long-term benefit and for the doctor's self-maintenance in safeguarding his freedom to be a full and autonomous human being.

In order to understand this process it may help to consider how it may have developed through childhood experience. Let me hypothesize about a child's upbringing, first as an infant and then as an older child. You may feel this is only theoretical, but bear with me and see if a useful picture develops.

Imagine, if you will, an infant with its mother. The infant is not well and is struggling to breathe. It coughs and splutters but then really does nearly choke on inhaled secretions. It feels ill; it senses that something is seriously wrong; it finds that it is needing to struggle to breathe and finds this dreadfully distressing. Suddenly there is a great build up of anxiety as breathing changes from being difficult, to near impossible, and choking intercedes. These are very unpleasant and frightening feelings. There is panic.

Now in our mind's eye, let us observe the mother. Let us assume she is a concerned and sensitive person. She therefore feels responsible for this small, poorly little being and knows her baby is distressed. From the baby she takes up the feelings of distress and anxiety for its safety as she observes its struggle to breathe. Then, as choking develops, fear and panic for life hooks into mother's growing concern for the baby. She perhaps turns her baby over and pats its back, holds it close and speaks soothingly to it. It is as if the baby's feelings and the mother's feelings and concerns are one. The baby's needs and the mother's concerns flow imperceptibly from baby to mother, who then translates them into the more effective actions of the adult. She thinks the situation through, sorts it out and finally, cradling baby quietly in her arms, hands back peace and calm – replacing the unpleasant feelings with pleasant ones. The sense of crisis is removed.

Now let us look to an older child. I recall a general situation when our youngest son returned from school with homework and was in a spin about it. He had to write two pages but he did not seem to understand anything more than this. I watched as my wife dealt with him. She, as it were, took on his anxiety and began working her way through it. 'Did the teacher make you write the question down?' 'It's in your book. Let's see.' 'Now what does it mean I wonder?' 'Well what were you learning about in the class?' 'So it was about birds. How do they feed their young?' etc., etc. By the end, our son clearly felt he knew what his homework was about, he had remembered that there was a chapter on it in his schoolbook, and was also clear that he had some ideas that he could write about from what he already knew of the subject. He could now deal with his anxiety himself and was able to work with it because he now understood and had it all in proportion.

Here again is an instance of a young person's intense anxiety being shovelled onto his mother. She quietly accepted it, was not overloaded into panic by it and helped him by first understanding it herself, then getting it into proportion and finally handing it back to the child in a manageable form. Such processes are clearly everyday ones in a child's experience. The frequency of the process makes it second nature to children (Bion, 1959).

These scenarios are common to all children and so there is in each person's background this frequent experience of handing over the unpleasant feelings they cannot manage to a receptive person. Note that in childhood it will usually be with a parent or parental figure that this process of projection will take place. Not surprisingly then, adult patients may unwittingly continue to use a parental or authority figure as the recipient of their projections. This is especially so at times of crisis, such as illness, when they are once again dependent on an authority figure. The doctor is therefore especially likely to receive strong projections. With increasing maturity the individual progressively recognizes the whole range of his feelings and can more readily accept them for what they are, and does not need, so frequently or heavily, to use others in this way.

But not all children have understanding adults around them. What happens when a child's projected feelings are not accepted or acceptable to the parent and are not therefore accepted or given validity by the process already described? The child is left with a serious dilemma. For instance, he may hear 'Don't you stamp your foot at me' or, 'Big boys don't cry'. In these circumstances he does not experience the sharing and mutual understanding of his angry or hurt feelings that would enable him to own, value and use them. Instead he learns to deny those feelings and he will continue to free himself of them by projection, right into, and possibly throughout, his adult life.

These are familiar enough scenarios. It can be deduced from them that 'projectors' are likely to be people who have not had their bad, angry, anxious selves responded to with acceptance; and, because they have not had non-judgemental help to integrate their difficult feelings when they were children and rightly dependent, they must now continue to project or 'split' (Klein, 1952) them off from themselves. By this splitting process, the judgemental projector is, in the short term, enabled to keep some sense of good opinion about himself but at the cost to someone else of carrying his difficult feelings.

What feelings may be projected? It has been noted that they would be the type of feelings that for various reasons are unwanted and too uncomfortable to hold onto oneself. They might include anger, frustration, fear, humiliation, powerlessness, confusion, madness, emptiness, anguish, despair, sexuality and so on: all the feelings that the parents found difficult or unacceptable.

Projection is an everyday experience: it is subtly and unconsciously happening all the time. It is frequently a first resort when people suddenly find themselves overcome with feeling. Although unconscious, it forms part of human communication. When healthy, the adult projector will, within a short period of time, become able to own his feelings for himself and they are then no longer projected. This process of taking ownership and full responsibility for oneself is helped by talking about incidents and their resulting effects on the inner world of the person. What is less healthy is when it is long denied and firmly placed on others. Unwanted and denied by the projector, and deposited on – rather than rooted in –

the recipient, they seem to have a power of their own. Because they remain hidden from consciousness, the recipient cannot work to an understanding of them nor do anything with them, unless he has some knowledge and experience of the projection process. The unconscious nature of the interaction gives it a quality of the unseen and the mysterious, so that a feeling of the magical or of confusion may make him unsure of himself. While it stays unconscious and unknown its power remains.

Mario Jacoby, in his book, *The Analytic Encounter* (1984), gives a diagram adapted from one of Jung's drawings and I further adapt it here to elucidate this process.

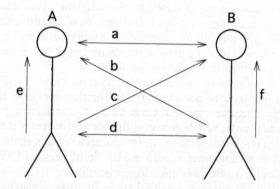

Figure 1 *Figure to elucidate the text in relation to conscious and unconscious communication*

Adults often communicate by talking. This conscious communication is represented in the diagram by the line drawn between the heads of the two stick men, A and B.

There may also be other communications that are recognized only by one person. So, for instance, person A may give out unconscious messages of being low and depressed. These may be through his slow speech delivered in a monotone, or he may look sad, hold his shoulders hunched, be grossly overweight, and his face, hands and voice may show no animation. He is not conscious of his feelings but the observer is. Such communication from one person's unconscious to the other's conscious self, are represented by the lines b and c and represent one person's unconscious feelings that are understood and consciously known by the other. Then there is line d. This represents feelings that are being unconsciously rejected, split off, projected and picked up by the other person equally unconsciously. For instance, any depressed body-language of person A in the diagram, if not consciously understood by person B, could, nevertheless, be unconsciously pick up by B and affect his reaction to A. The unconscious, unknowing aspect of this communication means that there is a mystifying, intuitive element to the process. Neither is aware of the communication, only that they find themselves mysteriously able to react one with the other. Note that it is possible for each to learn to make these processes available to their conscious selves so that they become aware of them, (represented by the lines e and f).

There are useful discussions about projection in many analytic and psychotherapy books. *Object Relations Therapy* by Sheldon Cashdan (1988) is one that is fairly clear and succinct.

The concept and implications of projection can be difficult to fully grasp and use. Those studying to become psychotherapists, and who are therefore working to understand and use this central plank for their work, will often understand it with their heads long before they can grasp it to the point where they can perceive and define the feelings they have received in this way and begin to use the process. People who do break through the learning barrier and both assimilate the ideas and develop an ability to apply them have an immensely useful tool in communication. Once the process is recognized, the frequency with which it occurs and the ramifications of its effects can begin to be appreciated.

The theory of projection can help a doctor in various ways. For instance, if he finds himself feeling angry when he is with a patient, it can be difficult to understand why and so be able to contain or hold onto the angry feeling so as to use it beneficially, but with this concept of projection he can analyse the situation and, understanding himself, be in a position to do something with the anger.

For example, when a doctor feels angry in a consultation with a patient, he can ask himself; 'Have I a reason to be feeling angry?' He is perhaps aware that the patient was a few minutes late but that would not normally bother him too much. He may recall that a telephone call earlier had annoyed him, but he has already worked out what he is going to do about that, and plans to talk it through later in the day with the person concerned. That, too, would not be disrupting his feelings as much as this. He may then surmise that the smiling patient who sits in the chair in front of him is in fact projecting her anger onto him. Even just understanding this possibility can make the anger become less personal and less heavy, and as a result it becomes more manageable. He is also now in a position to try checking out if it is indeed the patient's anger, and to have a go at handing it back.

He is freeing himself to some degree to be able to work with what is going on, and to shed a sense of impotent acceptance. He might say, for instance, 'I suspect you are feeling annoyed at the situation you find yourself in', and if the patient acknowledges she is, he can explore this with her and will find the anger in himself subsides when it becomes owned by the patient. The patient's anger, and its focus, can now become clear to them both.

Of course the patient may not be ready or able to own her feeling and it may take more than one question to encourage her to take the unwanted feeling back, but these are skills the doctor can develop and so improve the outcome.

It should be clear from this description of a doctor/patient interaction that an important element of what the patient was talking about had not been given verbal recognition by the patient, but it had nevertheless been communicated to her doctor by projection. This feeling element of her communication was, in this instance, verbally acknowledged by him and the patient could then be made aware of the communication, as well as discover her own feeling. Therefore, besides this being an example of the handling of her projection, it is also an example of the doctor listening to his patient in the fullest possible way. As such it can give a patient considerable satisfaction and a sense of being well understood. At the same time, the doctor has pleasure in the interaction because it has due depth and gives them both satisfying rapport. It is an example of a most intimate and full communication despite the inauspicious start to their interaction. However, the reality is that it is hard and skilled work to get a person who projects to take back their feeling and own it. Indeed, unless the projector is on the verge of being conscious of their feelings, it is unlikely that, in an ordinary consultation, a doctor will be able to move patients into being fully aware of them. Just as in the case of the business woman who demanded a hysterectomy, quoted at the start of this chapter, a doctor can often only hope to maintain himself and hold onto his integrity as a person. A more full and satisfying relationship is unlikely.

Another example of projection taken from a family practice setting, and which involves the projection of quite a different feeling, will help develop the concept as well as serve as an illustration of the all-pervasive frequency of the process.

A man used to come regularly to his doctor for blood pressure treatment and always seemed friendly and warm. Towards the end of what was usually a shortish consultation, he would ask after the doctor's children: 'What were they doing?' 'Were they still at home?' While in some ways this seemed to be in context with this man's warm friendliness, and yet, as the doctor acknowledged to himself, he did have a photo of his family beside his desk, but other patients did not usually ask after his family if they did not know them. Over a period of time the doctor found himself giving more and more information, just a bit here and there. But he also noticed that each time, after the patient had left, he was uncomfortable and disturbed. He found he did not look forward to seeing this particular patient and he had a sense that his doctoring was not adequate even though the patient's medical condition and its treatment were straightforward. He felt confused as, on the one hand, there was this open, warm and friendly patient with an easily treated medical condition and, on the other, he was uncomfortable with each consultation.

Eventually his interest in his own disquiet made the doctor look into what was happening. 'You are always so interested in my family,' he said in a questioning way (as this was the most obvious different behaviour he had noted). It then became clear that after World War II, while away in the army, the patient had had a son but had not kept in touch with the mother and he did not have any knowledge of the whereabouts of his child who would now be a man. He had returned home and married a local girl, but he and his wife had had no children. There was much sorrow and sadness here. But other patients have similar distresses in their lives and the doctor had not found himself personally dispirited by contact with them.

Dr Joseph Berke describes the grasping, emptying, scooping-out effects of envy. There is destruction of what is good, and feelings of emptiness, uselessness and loss of pleasure in the recipient (1984). Armed with this knowledge, the doctor began to see that his own distress with the consultations had probably been as a result of a projection by the patient and resulted from an envious grasping of the doctor's good feelings. Just that understanding alone enabled a change in the doctor so that the patient's feeling could be voiced, and in their later discussions the patient spoke of his lost son with longing and it became apparent that he did indeed envy the doctor his family and the contacts he had with them. Once this was out in the open, a shift for the better in their relationship then followed. The patient began to own his feelings so that they no longer remained deposited in the doctor. The patient became a more wholly aware and responsible person, and the contacts between patient and doctor became more real, losing their unpleasant undertone.

I suspect a dispirited doctor will frequently be one who has succumbed to projections of malice – but more of this in subsequent chapters.

CHAPTER 8

Patterns of Projection

There are many different feelings and each can be projected but, because of the nature of their work, doctors are particularly vulnerable to some of them. This chapter explores a small selection: the projections of dependency, sexuality, impotence and stress, and also projection occurring during telephone conversations and by people in groups.

So far projection has been described as being of a single feeling. However, as might be expected, there are variations to that simple model and the projection of dependency is one of them. It is as though, with dependency, rather than just one feeling being involved, there is the projection of a whole way of relating. The interaction can probably best be conveyed by saying that it is as if the doctor is drawn into experiencing the patient as a small, unprotected, powerless and totally dependent child, while he himself feels compelled to respond by being a totally dependable parent. It is as though the patient is a defenceless child hanging onto the doctor with its arms around his neck and somehow in fear of its life and for whom the doctor alone can be a saviour. It is as though, without the doctor's assistance, the patient would be alone and defenceless in a threatening world, frail, and quite unable to cope, while the doctor may have a sense of there being some imminent calamity, and feel himself to be hugely responsible. He may later muse on how it was that he gave far more of his time, and devoted more of both his physical and emotional energy on this patient's behalf than he could justify in retrospect. He may be left feeling anxious that he has indeed failed in his duty to the patient: for example, feeling concerned that something he has said, which was quite trivial in itself, will have been far too hard on the patient so that he believes he has jeopardized the relationship on which this patient is so very dependent. It is as if he is 'his' patient's only life-line, both physically and emotionally.

Sally had four children. Her husband was a labourer and they had little money for extras such as a car. She felt distressed by her life and presented a picture of helplessness. She was trapped, she said, by a small family income, her young children and a husband who, when not working, would go to watch football or go fishing. She felt she had to stop at home to cook, clean and take care of the family.

There was, she said, nothing else she could do. Her pleading eyes and impotent distress screamed for compassion as she requested that her doctor tell her what to do. Her sense of entrapment and helplessness led her to feelings of suicide that further increased the pressure and urgency on her doctor to do something. He, in his turn, felt her hopelessness and anxiety, but he had learned enough to know that her real need was to make adjustments within herself; so he limited himself to holding the feelings of distress, slowly enabling her to explore them for herself, and firmly grasped his role as her doctor, rather than act as good neighbour.

In succeeding weeks he was to hear that her own mother had been a helpless person and, on her death, when Sally was only ten, it was apparent that her father had felt relieved of the burden of caring for his wife. However, the father himself then took on the role of being helplessly dependent, so that Sally, his oldest daughter, was not only caring for her brothers and sisters but also pressured into taking care of him. Both her parents had therefore acted out the message: 'If you love me, you take care of me', while she had herself experienced little love and care. When she married she had become helpless in her turn so as to draw that same sort of love and care from her husband. This was not thought out: it was quite unconscious. He, however, was now breaking out of the 'I'll take care of you' mould, and she needed to discover both a different way of relating and how to be free to be herself. This seemed to be the crux of her long-term need. Her doctor explored with her what she did to spoil herself. There seemed to be nothing. 'What in your wildest dreams would you want for yourself?' She did not know. 'It sounds as if you need to discover what you want for yourself so that you can give it to yourself or arrange for it.' With time she agreed to go to see a counsellor, electing to spend some of her scarce money on herself to see if she could discover what she wanted.

It was really important if this woman's projection pattern was to be altered that her doctor did not succumb to his strong feelings that he must be active on her behalf, and instead hold tight to the fact that she was a fully grown, physically fit woman, able to order her own life. But he did not find this easy in the face of her powerful projection of dependency.

Developmentally, all human beings go through a stage of life in which they are dependent and unable to be responsible for themselves, but as they mature they progressively become able to take their own responsibility. Of course, some will do so more slowly than others, and some may revert, for instance at particularly stressful times.

Degrees of dependency vary widely and some aspects of it are more obvious than others. One form that is disguised may be noted when the individual clearly has energy and works and functions well but, on more careful observation, can be seen not to make his own decisions, functioning only within a framework that has been given him. There are times when everyone needs to be able to do this, but what indicates this dependency is when there is an invariable inability to function without being given a framework. This inability may be hidden in patients who come to see their doctor again and again. It is as if they are saying, 'Tell me what to do and I'll go and do it', but they do not themselves take on the responsibility to work out their options and then make a choice. In these people the doctor may have a sense of the patient being stuck and of a passivity that is cloying and quite depressing. The patients themselves may then be seen to be defending against their depressed feelings by hyperactivity in some other area of life, as if in an attempt to cover up their depression and to compensate. However, their localized hyperactivity only serves to maintain the status quo and, one way or another, the doctor can feel dispirited by the patient's distressing situation and wearied by the concern he holds for them and the extra effort he makes on their behalf.

Most doctors take a pride in not letting their patients down and in being dependable, so that it is easy for them to be sucked into doing what dependent people want. The doctor becomes important to them. They say such things as: 'Oh thank you, doctor. I really do not know what I would do without you.' They tell their friends, and they, too, then come to swell the list of people who think the doctor wonderful. His pedestal grows, consulting hours lengthen, patients wait for him to return from his holidays. He really is a popular doctor. His spouse, of course, is fed up with his work. (It would be more accurate to say that she is fed up with her husband.) He tires as he works to polish up his image by doing more and more for these people, but he is not a free person and is caught up in projections of dependency that have hooked into him and which deplete his energy and effectiveness.

Another projection pattern that is particularly relevant to family doctors is that of sexuality. Once again this is probably best thought of as the projection of a type of relationship rather than simply of just one feeling. A presentable young woman had always struck her doctor as being coy. During one consultation with her he had a feeling that she had something very special that he did not. She alluded to situations that spoke of fun, and which she clearly considered were very important to her. It seemed they were rarely to be found, but enabled a fullness of experience. It began to dawn on the doctor that these situations were sexual experiences. Only with an effort of mind did he recall that she had overtly come to talk about her difficult relationship with her husband who, she claimed, was madly jealous. He found himself feeling both curious about what sexual experiences she might be alluding to, and also feeling that his own experience must be insufficient and inadequate by comparison. Curiosity grew to arousal, and a need and desire to prove his full sexual powers, perceiving them as otherwise curtailed in some way. It was as if nothing else seemed to matter: sex overshadowed everything. His feelings burnt up into a fire that threatened to overpower his thought processes – with their ability to inform him of what he had and valued at home and which would, at least in part, be lost and devalued if he followed the feelings of the moment. His physical being, unbridled by the numbing of his thought processes, yearned to be drawn in. He was caught in a strong projection of sexuality, and the patient's subsequent seductive behaviour (which included making appointments to see her doctor so as to be the last patient at night, and making late-night requests for visits for 'severe chest pains' and 'low abdominal pains' to an otherwise empty house) added to the picture and strength of her projection.

It was important for the patient and her relationships, and for the doctor and his family, that he regain his own power and unfreeze his thought processes so as to give counterbalance to the power of feelings. The doctor must draw on his store of empathy for the patient and remind himself that the patient's personality must be severely wounded for her to act as she does, a wound that his own involvement would only serve to deepen (Rutter, 1990). He can remind himself that she is bringing that pathology to him in his professional capacity, and that she is not drawn to him because of romantic feelings for him as a person. He is helped by reminding himself of his self-value and by clarifying what he wants and values at home and, for instance, of his reasons for becoming a doctor – a position he risks losing.

In these situations a doctor can be greatly helped by an understanding of the theories of interpersonal processes and the real need and disability of the patient. In the above example it was to transpire that the patient's strong projections resulted from a sense in her that she was not desirable or of value except sexually. Other than sexually she was empty and deeply sad. She existed for sex and to ensnare her numerous acquaintances. Entanglements fuelled her husband's jealousy which, in a superficial way, satisfied her need to be valued. Unconsciously she had brought her problems in the form of her behaviour to her doctor because they had their origins in a time when she did not have the words to describe what went on in her. Seen in this way it was as if she now acted them out as a demonstration, hoping for her doctor's professional help to free her from the grip of her destructive, repetitive behaviour.

Sexual involvement between a doctor and patient, and indeed between other caring professionals and their clients, is receiving growing recognition. Research undertaken in a variety of countries indicates that over 50 per cent of both male and female doctors admit to being sexually attracted to their patients, and that 10 per cent of male doctors admit to a sexual relationship (B.M.J., 1992). While, therefore, it is by no means uncommon, each instance is a source of major misfortune with powerful and degrading forces locking both participants together. Only by resisting the force of this projection can the patient's behaviour be discussed and used for healing – the reason why the patient has actually come, and the reason that the doctor has set himself up in his profession.

It is worth briefly generalizing about this. In these circumstances the patient's need is to free herself from a repetitive, compulsive, driven existence, so as to become able to relate as and when she wishes, and in a way that is appropriate and constructive in her life. She has turned trustingly to her doctor because of his role of healer. If he allows himself to participate and join in with the patient's demonstration of her difficulty, he serves only to enhance her problem by his abuse of her trust and of the position of power that her trust has handed to him. A door she had hoped would open to healing is closed in her face. The damage must surely be akin to that in the trusting daughter whose personality is warped for life by an abusing father, and to the father's damage that makes him unable to hold back from abusing her.

Women doctors also have the same problem with their patients of the opposite sex and homosexual men and women with patients of the same sex, though I find it difficult to imagine my way into these situations. Nevertheless they occur, and whether it is a male or female doctor, it does no service for the strength of feeling and the reality of the predicament not to acknowledge it. I understand that the doctors' professional bodies, and certainly a doctor's colleagues, invariably tend to conspire to defend the majority of their members. No one finds it easy, but what is needed is to sort these things through in a way, and to a point, that does justice to the long-term damage caused to the patient and the difficulty the doctor will otherwise surely get into again.

A third common projection pattern is that of psychological impotence. This projection is different in that so often the patient will free himself of his unacceptable feeling by projection, while at the same time hold to himself the opposite types of behaviour to an excessive degree. He projects feelings of inferiority, ineffectiveness and inability, and simultaneously clings to an image of great power and control by exercising dominating and heavily controlling behaviour which can suck those around him into being even more impotent and dependent. Within society, control and power are frequently seen as worthwhile objectives that are to be respected but, in reality, society's managers and leaders are too often people with an excessive need to control, as otherwise they do not feel safe and would be closer to an awareness of their own impotence. Of course, doctors, too, may have chosen their career because of their need for power and control, not just over death and pain, but also in an attempt to insure against an inner sense of disabling disaster or chaos.

A man came to his doctor to say that his son, Tom, had a problem. He often wet the bed, had asthma, got angry and was disrupting the family. The whole thing had come to a head because the son, now twelve years old, had shouted and sworn at his mother at the end of a church service. He was worried, he said, that Tom was developing bad habits and would not be 'a good Christian'. As they talked it seemed to the doctor that Tom was publicly blowing the whistle on his family, and so he told the father he needed to see all the family together. This was not practical, said father: his wife worked; he would bring his son. The doctor stood firm, saying that the whole family seemed to be disrupted and he needed to understand from each of them how they were affected if he were to clearly understand and be in a position to help. Eventually, despite powerful pressure from the father for the doctor just to tell him what he should do to his son, they all came.

Coming into the room each was told by father where to sit, and the children were told they must be still and quiet. Father did the talking, and when the doctor managed to get a question in, even when this was directed by name to an individual member of the family, father would answer for them. After the doctor had clarified with father that he needed to be able to speak to them individually and directly, father then took to asking one of his sons, or his wife (whichever it was that had been spoken to by name), if they had understood what had been said, and then told them to answer. He seemed to want to be the conductor of an orchestra, and to need massive control.

Repeatedly father reiterated the message that Tom had a problem with bed wetting, asthma attacks and with his temper. He had tried physical punishment and punishment by deprivation, and yet, he complained, his son only got worse. Finally he said in exasperation: 'he is uncontrollable and useless.'

The doctor's feelings at the time are of interest. He found this man offensively pushing and amazingly controlling. He felt himself to be quite useless and powerless, and really had to put a lot of work into just existing. He felt he did not want to be there with the man; it was too unpleasant; it was as if he could hardly exist in his presence except by being very determined, almost fighting, to hold his line. Everything he said or did was altered, changed, and made as nothing. It was stifling. He felt that if he had had a tendency to asthma, then this would have caused an attack. He felt he was experiencing the hemmed in, claustrophobic, stifling, impossible feelings the son knew so well.

The doctor now told them all that they as a family had a problem and that he needed to see them together several times to work with them. He told them that Tom was very helpful to the family in making it clear to everyone that there was a problem; and he set the family exercises in listening to each other as a way of challenging the father's implicit perception that only he had anything that was worth saying, and so as to allow them to spread their individual wings a bit while with each other. It was really hard to gain agreement from father for this, and the doctor could only get that agreement by maintaining that there was no other option for them and that he was sure the situation in the family would become worse unless they agreed to what he was advising.

He was to find that all the family were subjected to endless criticism and always with an underlying theme that they were incompetent and only would, or could, do things if overseen by father. They were pressured into doing what father considered was important, and to do it in the way that he considered was right. The whole was overlaid with father's certainty that 'Christian' principles and concerns (all undefined) were right and needed both instilling and constant checking. It was as if otherwise there would be a helpless slipping down some steep slope to – it was not clear where – but certainly into some terrible pit.

It was as if father felt he could exist as a person only if he had iron control of himself and the people around him. Control was everything. Later the doctor was to learn that this man's father and mother had argued endlessly. As a boy he had had to spend a lot of time with his mother who had continued to demand his care and attention well into his forties. This pressure had been reinforced by recurrent threats to commit suicide. She had often told him (the first time being when he was a child) that her life was not worth living because of her husband's anger. As a child he had felt panic at what seemed an inevitable breakup of his small world, as father's anger broke out time and again. He felt panic, but as a child he was pathetically impotent in the situation. Steadily he began to feel he had to relieve mother of his father's angry, argumentative stance in an attempt to control his mother's suicidal threats and safeguard his own childhood world. By controlling his own feelings of desperate panic, and by constantly attempting to control the family situation, he learnt to make his life seem possible. No wonder the doctor had experienced him as exercising iron control and that everyone around this patient was made to feel incompetent and impotent. No wonder the doctor had to react firmly to hold onto himself as a person and work hard to be effective in this man's presence. The way out for the man and for his son was for him to find that now, as an adult, he would be all right when others were not under his control, and that his own feelings had importance and could similarly be given free rein. It would take time, but it was urgently needed for the son, the family and for himself.

The power of this projection, to suck the doctor into the patient's way of being, was enormous. Coming at the doctor in a pincer movement were the man's unconsciously made assumptions of his doctor's impotence and also, as a further defence, the man's own display of an apparently great competence and power. It needed considerable effort by the doctor to keep himself as a person with his own needs, wishes, values, and any sense of his own ability. He felt anger whenever he was sucked into not being himself. He had to acknowledge and value his anger in order to be able to maintain himself if he was to stand any chance of being effective with the family. Even describing the situation years after the event, the doctor found himself flattened and disturbed.

This is an especially strong example of the projection of impotence although it is suffused with other projected feelings, too. It is a common projection for doctors to field. Patients may comment on the doctor's youth, ask in a disparaging way which medical school he trained at, ask if he has much experience of their particular problem, and so forth. Yet it is the doctor's feelings of inability and uselessness in the face of this that must alert him to the projection. He can then hold onto his knowledge, skill and experience, to combat the projected feeling.

Projections are difficult and stressful to handle, but as well as being stressful to the recipient, stress itself can be projected. It is worthwhile considering the projection of stress separately.

A doctor may well be feeling his own stress because of his clinical responsibilities, but on top of this he can then be heavily loaded by the patient's projected stress. Once again, the patient's projected feeling cannot be directly understood and managed by the doctor as it does not originate in him and it is not therefore in his power to understand. Meanwhile, his feeling of being stressed can overload him and may prevent him working through those stressful feelings which are his own.

This can be extremely discomforting and, of course, unmanageable stress will result in some people turning to drugs, such as nicotine or alcohol, to calm themselves. They become dependent on drugs instead of discovering how to cope with the factors that have produced the stress, or of understanding the processes of projection. Unfortunately, by not themselves taking responsibility to sort out the feeling and make adjustments accordingly (but instead, relying on a drug of some kind) they progressively lose their coping skills rather than developing them to keep pace with increasing maturity and life experience. The result is increased reliance and addiction to their artificial prop.

The ricocheting effect of the projection of feeling is therefore especially obvious in relation to projected stress. Stress blinkers people and prevents them from adapting. Stressed people tend to develop tight systems and to proceed in straight lines. They have no free energy to consider what may lie to left and right and, as a result, cut out much of what makes life rich and interesting. They often attempt to impose their 'efficiency' on the people around them, pressing their family and colleagues into the same straight-line ways of being, or tight systems of organization, which threaten their freedom to be whole people. Happily, most people do not accept tight systems for long, reacting to the projected stress and the imposed stressful situations by breaking out to reaffirm their humanity.

Highly stressed people are uncomfortable within themselves and will frequently envy those who are able to resist the pressure to join them in their highly stressed state. Their envy seeks to take away other people's good feelings about themselves, and to undermine their sense of self-worth. They treat others as if they have no existence of their own and as if they have no importance except to deliver whatever the projector chooses is important. The stressed person's own need and emptiness lies hidden beneath the surface.

And if they get what they want out of those around them, they will still not be satisfied. The more others try to accommodate them, the more it emphasizes their inherent emptiness. When one is confronted by stressed and envious people, the understanding of this model of projection can be very helpful in maintaining one's own separate existence. Often, however, people's untutored reaction to this sort of extreme pressure is either to join in with the projector's wishes or to take an opposite and equally extreme stance. The trick is to remain oneself and be as you yourself wish to be, neither sucked in, nor overly reacting against the pressure.

It is worth briefly considering the inner world of people who habitually project their feelings. Imagine, if you will, a person with many feelings that are not acceptable to him and so are projected. He is left, therefore, not sure what he feels, and because he is unsure of himself he becomes highly anxious, and must rely on others. But his anxiety, too, may be too great to bear, so that this feeling is also projected. From this ill-functioning position, he looks around and sees others who seem free to be themselves, so that envy can be added to the load of uncomfortable feelings which he may also find unacceptable and therefore projects in its turn. This endlessly spiralling picture of a succession of unbearable feelings, each projected one after the other, results in the individual being left confused as to who he is and what, deep down, he really wants to be. It is a distressing picture which unfortunately is the internal state of a significant number of people who come to their doctors.

So far this chapter has only considered projections between individuals who meet face to face, but projection of feeling is also relevant in telephone conversations. Knowing this can be helpful when seeking to utilize the telephone to best advantage. Projections are strongest when communication is incomplete and when, as a result, assumptions abound. Under normal face-to-face conditions people make considerable use of visual signals, such as facial expressions and hand gestures to fill out the total picture. These are used to aid the development of trust in what is being said (Frank, 1991). In general, doctors are especially aware of body language, using it to form a more secure picture of what patients are saying about their illnesses. However, when the telephone is being used these physical indicators must either be abandoned or replaced by words. Doctors are usually only trained in face-to-face consultations and yet this change in circumstance requires thought, practice and extra effort, otherwise assumptions will result and, if not checked out, will often form projections. For instance, with 'urgent' out of hours' telephone calls, patients are usually anxious and are telephoning in the hope of relieving themselves of their anxiety. Where, for instance, they are fearful for life, that anxiety can be unbearably strong, and as a result will often be projected onto the doctor at the other end of the telephone line. The patient may assume that the doctor will find their condition one that causes him just as much anxiety as it does them, and this projected assumption, left unexplored, may make a doctor visit when, with more full communication, there would have been no need. What encourages this process is that doctors are so often trained to consider only the patient's physical body. If patients are not considered holistically, and are held to have no ability to monitor and reflect on themselves, a doctor may, like doubting Thomas, have a strong need to see the physical body if he is to have faith that a patient can be all right, and therefore he must make a visit to their homes.

The subject of telephoned 'urgent' requests for visits was discussed in Chapter 4. That chapter explored one way in which the telephoned projection of anxiety can be turned around so that, rather than cause undue pressure, it becomes a useful tool for the doctor. The level of the patient's projected anxiety is thereby used to monitor the effectiveness of the doctor's telephone work and he can become more able to assess accurately when it is necessary to visit. As a result telephone skills are refined for the greater comfort of all concerned.

There is another important variation of circumstance where projection often occurs and which certainly affects doctors. It forms another whole area of interest and lies within the realm of group dynamics. A group of people may join in splitting off unwanted feelings and project them onto an individual or onto another group.

Recently I was involved in a working conference of doctors where the work was done mostly in two groups. One group chose to focus on a detailed plan for some future activity and, at the plenary session at the end of the conference, they were brimming with excitement and full of their ideas. The second group, however, had chosen to explore the difficulties of their job and the uncomfortable and distressing parts of their work. Rather than plan ahead, they chose to share and understand each other's difficulties. At the plenary session their spokesperson therefore reported their vulnerability and struggle.

At this point in the plenary session many in the first group – the excited planning group – saw themselves as having been a 'good' group, and also talked of the other group as having had an unfortunate experience and judged that it had been a 'bad' group. Not only were the feelings of the second group seen as difficult, but the group was not felt to be acceptable either. People who could allow such feelings had been labelled 'bad'. It was as if people's 'dangerous' feelings must be kept under control or the group's members must surely have failed. Here was a denial of the whole person, but this time by a group of individuals. It is an example of the process of projection occurring between groups, and is part of the process of making others into scapegoats.

I will give another group example to show projection's multitude of guises in group situations and to underline both how common it is and its relevance to doctors. In a partnership one doctor may be particularly sensitive to depressed feelings and less able than his colleagues to defend against other people's depression. The group may then dump its depressed feelings onto that member, even to the extent that he becomes ill. If such a dynamic is relentless and not understood, such a member may actually have to leave the partnership in order to regain freedom to hold only his own feelings. Meanwhile, of course, the rest of the group must look for another person on whom to dump their depression, or hopefully they may develop the ability to own it themselves.

Group behaviours such as these occur in families, in partnerships and between organizations – all situations affecting doctors. There are extreme forces at work in projection and they can bend and take control of other people's lives. They are a source of major discomfort for doctors, threatening their freedom to be persons in their own right.

The family doctor is not working with a representative group of people from the population. Distressed, malfunctioning people are the norm in the consulting room. Estimates vary of the percentage of people with mainly psychological problems who attend their doctor, but as has already been pointed out, Dr Michael Balint (1957) considered this to be more than 40 per cent, though others have given much higher figures. Certainly a significant amount of the doctor's work is with people who, to some degree, are psychologically distressed and, of course, these people attend again and again. Not surprisingly, then, the doctor is subjected to one projection after another and commonly he may have several strong projection experiences in just one morning of consultations. Projections are largely of unpleasant feelings and a doctor carrying them, particularly if the process is not understood, will experience them as a heavy load. In such circumstances it is easy for a doctor to give up the struggle of maintaining himself, but to do so will inevitably mean going under and losing his sense of self.

CHAPTER 9

The Distressed Patient

After a general discussion this chapter will draw on two examples of
distressed patients to demonstrate how the same predominant feeling can produce quite different situations for the doctor. Super-
ficially, each example appears to exhibit a very different picture but,
at a deeper level and with the concept of projection in mind, they
can be seen to be fundamentally the same.

Generally speaking, doctors are people who want to be active
in helping others. If someone is in physical pain then they rightly
relieve it or refer on to someone who can. What, though, of the
patient distressed by the psychological pain of one of life's many
adversities? What is the doctor to do in those situations? Where,
if at all, does his activity lie? What is his responsibility?

For example, when a woman's husband is reported to have
suddenly and unexpectedly died, what is there to do? I am clear
the doctor does a great deal by daring to be with her; by not, as
it were, crossing over the road to the other side, but by staying
and thereby saying: 'I will share this moment with you; I will
support you; I will listen to your sobs or your anguished words; I
will be with you in your silence, or as you speak your pain.' This
alone is valuable.

It may be that a doctor will talk over some aspect of what is
going on, turning it over with his words and bringing greater
understanding to this pained person. The message is: 'It is worth
talking and sharing. You do not have to lock it up. It is part of
life. Experience this part of life and put it into words with me – if
not now, we can arrange another time.'

As the doctor cannot stay forever, and certainly cannot replace
the lost person, he can only establish that there needs to be
someone there for them to talk to when they wish, and then help
the patient to seek stepping stones of contact until she has
picked up her own friends and supports as they learn of her new
situation. He may judge that it is best if he himself is one of
those stepping stones for a short time, but it may be that he
already has his share of distressed people who talk with him (and
realistically he can only take on a share), or that he knows he has
too much on his plate just now, in which case the doctor's belief
in the need to share and talk, needs expression through an expec-

tation that the patient will need to make contact with someone else for this purpose. The widow who does not have the skill to talk, or friends to talk with, may need the offer of the telephone number of a counsellor.

A doctor's own needs when he experiences loss can be a great help to him in understanding what is needed in these situations. It was when speaking on the telephone to my brother that it became clear to me that he had a cancer secondary in his brain. It had suddenly affected him, and meant that he could not easily talk until I started the ball rolling; if I opened up a relevant subject, then he could follow on. We talked for, I do not know how long, thirty minutes I suppose. Slowly I was adjusting to what had happened and checking out this or that. He hung onto the conversation and to me. He found himself discovering his condition through our talking. Both of us needed this and both received a sense of each other's concern and love. My talking made him relax. It was as if I could slowly accept what had happened and what he now was, and handling it with words made it less unknown, less fearful, something that was not untouchable for both of us.

When I put the telephone down, then my distress flooded me. I cried out uncontrollably, and as the words formed they were, 'No, No, NO'. I needed to be alone for a short while just adjusting to his never being the same again and the realization that he was not going to be around for long. My need now was to cradle myself. A little later I needed to carry this deep, deep cry and this dreadful news and my distress, to share it with my wife, Ann. I needed nothing more from people. I needed to know the diagnosis; I needed time to myself; and I needed time with people to talk of what was happening in Bernard and then also in me; time for shared feelings. For some time afterwards, I needed to have time for these things. It meant free-wheeling with work and, while his condition became worse, a little time out of work as holiday. But there was nothing else I needed beside a mix of these commodities for as long as it took: nothing actually done for me.

It was noteworthy that over the months of my brother's illness, the most helpful people outside the family were two young doctors who, from time to time, perhaps over a pub meal, would ask what was happening to my brother. My brief initial replies were picked up by their asking further questions and encouraging me to explore with them. I found that what was happening in him and in me was apparently of concern to them, and they gave their reactions. For example, I remember the words, 'That's awful', giving me a great sense of being understood. What seemed to be most helpful was the sharing of feelings: feelings briefly shouldered by another; feelings better refined and understood through another's perceptions; feelings that, when received back, were less heavy because of the experience of their having been briefly carried by a companion.

That being the case, the doctor offers patients a most valuable commodity when he gives them time. They may talk, or remain silent. He may sense they need him to talk sometimes, and at others, say nothing. They are sustained by his presence and at the end they go, knowing they can come again.

Often a distressed person will feel dreadfully alone and isolated. This one feeling of isolation or aloneness can in itself be immensely painful, and comes, of course, on top of the feelings of distress. As a result it can be strongly projected so that the doctor can hardly bear it. Nevertheless he need not be concerned at his need to leave. No problem. The patient is experiencing normal life. The doctor's life goes on, just as, with time, the patient will feel as if his life, too, is moving again. For the doctor to go is therefore just as reassuring as to come.

It is difficult when people seem persistently unable to talk. Many are not used to talking about their intimate problems. Some can only talk about things – work, a film, politics, a hobby. There are others who have entered a phase of being inturned. I think people like this have a problem believing that their inner world is of any value or importance, or they may not really be in touch with what goes on inside themselves anyway. They come into the room and the doctor can feel their distress: it is palpable. They desperately need to talk, and yet they cannot.

In my early days in family practice I was called by a confused mother to her thirteen-year-old daughter. I certainly was not clear why I was going and mother could only say her daughter was behaving strangely and looked frozen. I arrived to find she had been put to bed upstairs, and I found that she had obviously been crying, but was now silent. She seemed fearful and she certainly did look frozen. She filled me with a sense of horror, fear and shock, of not knowing, of isolation and loneliness. These feelings had a strength and quality that I had learnt were those of projected feelings; so she was communicating with me by projection, even though she was saying nothing. I would have to fly by the seat of my pants. I sat on the bed. What else did I know about her? She had moved into this house when her father had died. There were just the two of them, mother and daughter. The room was bare except for ill-fitting curtains, the bed and a hard chair. It was cold. I had my coat on and I buttoned it up. So they were having hard times. There was no man around the place for mother; no father with whom daughter could learn how to relate to men. This was in my early days in general practice and I had had no past experience that seemed to help.

I talked of what I knew, mirroring back to her what messages I did receive. 'It must be hard for you living here away from the friends and school you used to go to when you lived with Dad.' 'It must be hard to grow up with no father around, hard to do what you want when it means leaving Mum on her own.' 'I am feeling very cold: it must be shivery getting ready for bed.' 'I hope you are warm enough in there.' She began to relax and certainly she was listening and watching me intently. There was eye contact. We were engaging at some level and about something that was important to her. At one stage I held her hand and stroked it as I spoke. Here was further contact given and accepted. I left long silences, but she did not speak for the whole hour I was there.

At the end I told her that I thought she was shocked, distressed and fearful. I wanted to let her know I accepted her and told her, truthfully, that I liked her and was pleased her mother had called me. I told her that whatever it was that was going on in her, I felt it would be good to talk about it when she was ready, and that if she needed help in finding someone to talk to, then I could help find someone, or, if she wanted to talk to me, I would be there to listen. She had lost the strained and horrified look and could now manage a wan smile. I said, 'I need to go. Is that all right?' She nodded.

There are a lot of issues here, but this is an example of someone unable to communicate with words and yet in desperate distress and need of contact. I believe this because of the feelings that were projected into me of distress, isolation and intense loneliness.

Much later I learnt that this girl had been raped by a man whom both she and her mother trusted. She had indeed been filled with frozen horror, fear, and the loneliness that comes from trust misused. It is easy to speculate that in a person so young, her deeply disturbed feelings were likely to be too much to bear, and that she would need to project them if she was to retain her sense of self, rather than burst apart in an explosion of confusion and rage. I needed to be able to bear the strength and quality of her projected feelings. I was motivated by a belief in the value of the individual and the individual's right to call on another to be with them while they work through something in their own way.

Quite a different picture of distress was shown by a man of sixty-five when he came to see me for the first time. He had been to several opticians over the preceding months; all had prescribed yet a further pair of glasses, and he had found each pair unsatisfactory. He had become disillusioned. The long and the short of it was that he had now been operated on for a berry aneurysm, a swelling of a blood vessel in his skull which had pressed on the nerves to his eye, reducing his vision. The danger that this slowly stretching vessel would burst and kill him had necessitated an operation inside his skull and deep under his brain. While this had been life saving, it had also caused further permanent damage to his nerve tissue that resulted in an increased loss of sight and weakness in his hand. All this was in the past when he came to see me.

He was well able to speak his mind, and indeed it felt as if he would overwhelm me with his torrent of words, the strength of his feelings, and his huge stature. He had just begun to grasp that there would be little further improvement in his condition, and he was deeply distressed. Ever since he had been a teenager he had built up a collection of woodcarving tools, and in the past year he had erected a shed in his garden and made contacts with wood merchants, purchasing selected, well-seasoned pieces of hardwood, just right for the creations he had begun to plan. He had worked hard all his life and looked forward to contentment in creative retirement, but this had now been snatched away by this sudden illness. How could he carve when he could no longer see clearly enough? How could he handle his chisels with accuracy when his hand was weak and clumsy? He went into great detail and expressed his frustration openly and effectively. He knew his body had let him down and expressed his fury at his resulting disability and its timing. I doubt I could adequately convey the force and torrent of this man's detailed talk, and my feeling of being totally overwhelmed and inadequate.

The way this man presented himself at that interview would at first seem markedly different from that of the young girl. He came to see me of his own accord, while it had been the mother who initiated my contact with the girl. The man was very voluble, talking over his situation in great detail, while the girl had been totally passive. With her it had been me that was the active one, making the effort to go and see her, taking her hand in an effort to get in touch, doing the talking and putting two and two together in an attempt to understand. The man was overcome with distress and showed it by expressing it in every way he could and giving me something of his experience of being overwhelmed and impotent; while the girl was frozen with shock and a fear which she could not express nor cope with, and yet, through projection, she, too, gave me a sense of her inner experience of being frozen out. Both these people were overcome by their distress. They found it too much to bear and therefore they projected their feelings onto their doctor, even though each was outwardly behaving in quite different ways.

With both these patients there were other projected feelings beside their distress which also made the two consultations different, but nevertheless, these examples serve to illustrate several factors.

Apparently very different situations can be similar when looked at in depth. This would not be important in itself perhaps, except for what is, I believe, illustrated by these cases, and that is that all projections need broadly the same work by the doctor (Ogden, 1982).

Both situations were difficult and disturbing. In each the doctor needed to give the patient time and trust the process that the patient was going through. In that one long interview with the girl, and in a succession of short interviews with the man, the doctor was steadily used less and less to carry the patient's projections. Given time, both these patients progressively carried their own feelings more and more as they became less overwhelmed by them. They could integrate their feelings and become whole people once more. The main activity and the process were theirs and would, of course, continue between consultations.

These examples are both of a doctor working with distressed people but they are also examples of extremes. In the first there is distress resulting in an isolated patient with the doctor held at a distance. In the second, the doctor found himself swamped by the distressed patient who over-involved and overwhelmed him. The man flooded the doctor and gave him the experience of being enmeshed and ensnared. There is a continuous line, a continuum of different styles of relationship, with these extremes of isolation and over involvement at opposite ends, and between the extremes is the rich mix of the degrees of human involvements.

What is the norm? I doubt there is one, but I find that I myself sometimes need to be on my own and sometimes need intimacy. I need to be free to move from one to the other and to all places in between; to obtain the depth of intimacy and communication appropriate to myself, the situation and the person I am with at the time. The doctor can facilitate this flexibility in patients by his own flexibility in accepting where the patient is on any one occasion, and by helping them see their options by speaking of them as lying within their choice and attainment. He also holds the understanding that their present situation is only a phase. By drawing on wider dimensions of understanding, he can feed the patient's self-comprehension.

The doctor's activity is in observation, in understanding the situation, and in giving verbal feedback about these to the patient. His observations and understandings clarify and affirm what is happening within them, making it part of normal, expected life. His under-

A Doctor's Dilemma

standings come from what the patient says, from what he sees of the patient, from his knowledge of the norms of human personality development and behaviour, and from the insights resulting from the patient's projected feelings. Through the doctor's verbal reflections on all these, the patient can come to experience and know himself more fully, can come to hold his feelings for himself, and become more complete and secure. He will become more attuned to life and be a more effective person. But it is noteworthy that these understandings, and the doctor's ability to aid people to make these adjustments towards their wholeness, are greatly aided by a knowledge of the processes of projection. It is a fortunate side-effect that as the patient holds his own feelings more and more, the doctor is progressively freed from the stress of holding them on his behalf.

CHAPTER 10

The Doctor's Hook – The Part Played in Accepting a Projection

There are enormous implications for doctors in the concept of projection and the power of its processes to ensnare and stress them but it is possible for the doctor to hold a stance that makes him less vulnerable and he can take action to free himself from projection's power when it has occurred.

The previous chapters have outlined a process by which people project onto someone else who is more able to contain it, a feeling which they themselves find too difficult or frightening. It is as if the patient unconsciously casts out his unwanted feelings, like a fisherman with his rod, to hook into an unsuspecting recipient. Clearly all sorts of people can get 'caught' but here we happen to be considering doctors. Sometimes the cast will catch one doctor and sometimes another. What is it about an individual that enables a cast to take hold?

It is as if the doctor may also have a hook that makes him susceptible to being caught by the patient's projection. Some people have great big hooks, and some have hooks of lesser size. Some have hooks shaped to catch one feeling and others for another. Someone who is able to be angry will be available to pick up projected anger. Another, who can own his low, sad feelings, may be immune to projected anger, but will be a likely candidate for projected depression, and so on. It is as if the recipient will be someone who is able to identify with the feeling that is projected. If a doctor can be angry, a projecting patient may load him with his anger, just because the doctor is able to identify with it. It can also happen that the doctor becomes increasingly seen as an angry person. The patient can be all sweetness, but the doctor is left with all the sourness. Furthermore, the anger that the doctor experiences has an ungrounded character to it. Because it is not his own, he does not have access to the factors that have produced it; he does not know where it comes from, nor where he needs to focus in order to work with it. Frustration and confusion build up and may further increase the anger.

Whatever the size of the doctor's hook, and whatever the projection it seems shaped to catch, being caught is technically called projective identification. In this context, projection is what the patient does, and projective identification is what the doctor does when he identifies with the feeling and allows himself to assume it is relevant to himself; accepting it and taking it for his own.

This can probably best be explored through use of another example. Let us consider a projection that is particularly common in family practice and which is especially powerful because it fits so comfortably into the way many doctors perceive their role. As a result a doctor may readily assume the feeling to be his own and, accepting it as such, it is then difficult to spot, making it hard for a doctor to free himself from its power. It is also, I believe, frequently a source of much doctor over-commitment, and therefore a doubly potent stress-creator for himself and his family. It is the projection of 'ingratiation'.

I do not know how that word strikes you. Frankly, I initially found it smacked of something old-fashioned and unpleasant but I was not quite clear what it meant. One dictionary gives its meaning as, 'to win favour with'; another, 'to crawl, curry favour, fawn, flatter, grovel'. Here, though, its use is closest to the sense of 'winning favour', because the result of winning favour is the extra effort the recipient feels he must make if someone has 'earned' the right to a favour. Sheldon Cashden (1988) gives the process considerable clarity when he depicts the projector of in-gratiation as holding the attitude: 'I work extremely hard', with its underlying message: 'And you never do enough', resulting in the end point: 'so you owe me'.

The doctor's work is with the sick and disabled. Many of these people have a hard time compared to their healthy companions. They struggle and strain just to cope. They use up more energy and get more exhausted than the fit ones around them, and often for lower wages. They usually seem to have a less full and free life. They have been dealt an unfair hand. Do they not deserve better? If, on top of these reality factors, they are projecting the message: '... and you doctor, are fit and well, have a good life style with lots of interests and the money to pay for them – so you owe me.' It is very easy for the doctor to respond with: 'It is not their fault. I must go the second mile in my care of them.'

Here, the caring doctor can easily be sucked or hooked into working longer; doing more; stretching his finite resources of energy; and all because of his guilt at, for instance, being healthy, or at earning good money by comparison.

The facts are that the ill person is unlucky with regard to health, while the doctor is lucky enough to be fit and well. The doctor has to carry his feelings in relation to these uncomfortably juxtapositioned factors, which, when added to the nature of his job, intensify his desire to help care for those who are sick. But now add to this a projection of, 'So you owe me', and a doctor's hook of 'I *must* take care of you', will often result in the two becoming powerfully locked together.

The possibilities of this dynamic are scattered about almost everywhere in a doctor's work. For example, one of the difficulties many doctors have is of finishing a consultation at a reasonable time. Clearly it is not right to do so with a patient in extremis, but so often that is not the situation and yet patients can hold the doctor in the room, making him unable to draw the consultation to an end, unable to hold within himself the attitude, or indeed simply to say that their allotted, agreed time is up. This is often because of this underlying projected feeling that is met within the doctor by his agreeing, 'Yes, I do owe you'. The ingratiating patient may well have to make extra effort, is perhaps exhausted and tired, may be at the bottom of society's heap, and so can rightly draw the doctor's concern. The doctor may need to be an advocate on the patient's behalf with the caring agencies, or to blow the whistle on society's poor care of the underdog. However, he does not need to listen twice as long, or put in twice the effort that he makes with another patient who is perhaps more adversely affected and yet does not project 'You owe me'. The doctor needs to be free to be discerning, and to choose. He needs to be free from identifying with the projection, to be free to be himself and work appropriately to the patient's actual situation without internal coercion.

The processes of projection and projective identification can be looked at in reverse. For the purposes of this exercise, the doctor, as a result of his need to care for people, would be holding the attitude: 'I must look after you in order to feel good', and the patient the attitude: 'Yes, I need you to look after me as I am unable to care for myself and you owe it to me.' Seen in this way the doctor would be more whole if he either acknowledged his need to care, or freed himself from it, so that the patient in turn is free and challenged to be responsible and more fully himself.

Turning the example of the ingratiating patient around in this way is to see the doctor as projecting 'I *must* look after you; I need to be powerful and needed. I am more able than you. I have, and you have not. I can, and you cannot.' This clearly feels very unequal. It is as if the patient is not to be responsible for his own well-being, and as if the doctor has all the ability. The doctor denies his weakness, his vulnerability, his impotence and his struggle. These are the projections from which pedestals are built and smack of arrogance. They are set to hook another's debility and holds them in the position of being 'dis-abled' not only in body but also in mind and spirit; and meanwhile the doctor too is locked into a false perception of himself. Both the people involved defend against one set of feelings by covering them over with a preferred set.

Projection and the projective identification of ingratiation hide easily in the roles of patient and doctor and are common in the consulting room where it is especially invidious. The doctor is locked into a static, inappropriate, unreal world – but one to which he holds the key. Although at a superficial level patient and doctor may each like this situation, they are both stunted by it, and their development towards becoming full persons – each free and in charge of themselves – is halted. They cannot build on the firm foundations of reality. There is stalemate for them both. The patient's fundamental problems are not worked on, and the doctor holds a considerable frustration at their mutually inflexible, stuck and static state, along with the stress this engenders – and it is all to no good purpose.

The extreme and frequent result when projection has occurred will be one of two end points. The projected feelings are either accepted (when the two are then locked into projection and projective identification with both accepting the same view of their situation), or the recipient of the feelings is so disturbed by the strange package of projected feelings he receives that he strongly rejects it and the feelings boomerang back, making the projector not only again feel bad with his own feelings, but now also with the doctor's annoyance. But the end point in both these situations is that the projector is confirmed in his projective behaviour. In the first instance his projected feelings are accepted and he is free of them and, being unconscious of the process, feels comfortable and therefore will project again; in the latter situation, the feelings that are unacceptable to him are returned accompanied by the doctor's discomfort, and often experienced as if in a vengeful way. It is easy for the doctor to be blamed for this and blaming the doctor frees the projector from any dawning understanding of his own unhealthy processes, so that his need to project remains. But this has been to describe the two extreme, though common, end points of projection, and for the projector's behaviour to be changed requires reactions that are quite different to these. The work of treating people whose projective behaviour is deeply unconscious and firmly established falls into the sphere of the psychotherapist and analyst.

However, what can the doctor do when he has been hooked? There are a variety of things, and in general several or most of them will need to be used so as to gain his self-understanding and develop the boundaries of his personality until such time as he is used to the processes.

Certainly it helps to know of the theory and processes of projection as they provide a scaffold on which to build a clarity about what may be going on and to plan how to work accordingly.

It is necessary for the doctor to give time to reflect on his work. This is especially worthwhile when he is aware of feeling stuck, or is in some way ill at ease. Reflection time enables him to be more accurately aware of how he feels and to define his own state, as opposed to the feelings he experiences as a result of a patient's projections. He can then work out what those projections may mean for the patient, and plan effective ways to handle subsequent interviews to help the patient break out from his fixed behaviour and the doctor to find a similar freedom.

The process of projection may involve the use of words or maybe the patient is silent. Either way, the doctor, wishing to handle the situation differently, will need to work in such a way that the feelings are put into words. It is as if projecting patients make assumptions and do not check them out, but rather hold onto them, working as if their assumptions were an established reality. For example, a fairly frequent assumption by patients is that they have produced a problem that is for the doctor to sort out. This may be put into words: 'I am sorry to trouble you in this way doctor. I seem to have brought quite a problem for you.' A patient projecting his sense of discomfort at being stuck and unable to function may come with this spoken attitude. If the doctor does not accept their attitude (which holds him responsible for sorting the problem), and if he does not point this out, then from that point onwards, the two must function at odds with each other; clearly an unsatisfactory background for their work. If, on the other hand, this assumption is accepted by the doctor as if it were reality then it results in a feeling of pressure in him that he is likely to respond to by beginning to problem-solve on the patient's behalf. Often patients then play the 'game' 'Yes but' as described by Eric Berne in his book *Games People Play* (1968). Everything the doctor suggests is made out to have been tried adequately and to have failed totally, 'Yes but I've tried (something like) that and it doesn't work', or his ideas are held to be clearly not worth trying and discarded as of no value anyway and, as a result, the patient's attitudes are defended and not reconsidered. It is in ways like these that a doctor's sense of having a difficult problem is compounded and he can feel as stymied, impotent and frustrated as the projecting patient.

What is needed here is for the doctor to correct or challenge the patient's underlying assumption and give his own perception of the situation. It is the patient who has a problem; it is the patient who finds this difficult and who is unhappy with the situation as it is; and it is the patient who needs to find some other way of handling things if he is not to stay in his unhappy state. If the patient has difficulty taking this on board, it can be useful to emphasize this by saying at the end something like: 'I can see you feel stuck at the moment and will need to experiment further. It will be interesting to hear how you find a way to deal with your problem because it certainly can be satisfactorily resolved.' But one way or another, a clear understanding that the problem is the patient's produces a change in the background to the consultation that can free the doctor from the projection, and has a considerable baseline benefit for the patient.

Then there are projecting patients where the prevailing assumptions or attitudes are not spoken or alluded to. Perhaps these projections would be the most difficult to spot were it not that a doctor can be aware within himself of the patient's feelings. If he will allow himself to be aware of his feeling world, and will do the internal work of questioning and sorting them and, where necessary, checking them out with the patient, he becomes clear about the patient's inner world of assumption. This done, the doctor is ready, and once again will need to confront those perceptions and assumptions with words if he is to be free to be himself, and if he is to be of more use to the patient than merely to be used as a temporary dumping ground for unwanted feeling. An extreme example of this is the girl who had been raped described in the previous chapter. Her shock, distress and puzzlement were projected onto her doctor without any words being said about anything at all, let alone about her feeling state. Only by her doctor putting words to the feelings he experienced from her, could those feelings find any ownership in the girl. Both the girl and her doctor were then able to move on.

It can be useful to remind oneself that projection occurs as a normal phase in the pre-verbal young child, but the doctor is engaged in encouraging patients towards behaviour that is the norm in adults, and where the preferable, more accurate and most effective communication is through the use of verbal skills. The tools in dealing with projections are the adult abilities of being able to understand the process, of the open sharing of background attitudes, of the checking out of assumptions, of talking over the feelings involved and, as it were, inviting and encouraging the patient to acknowledge those feelings as being his own. To this end, a working knowledge of projection is a necessary background. The doctor can train himself to be aware of when the feelings he experiences are not his own, and then follow through these measures.

However, despite people's lives being enriched in the longer term by owning their feelings, in the short term they do not necessarily want to set aside their projection defence; something which would involve altering their preferred perceptions of themselves and of others. The doctor, working to free and extricate himself from the way a patient has long learnt to relate, will frequently be met with equally defensive, pressurizing anger. He will often be defensively blamed for this anger and must allow and accept this as inevitable. However, he will need to learn to be relaxed with angry people, and it will help him if he understands that the anger is a further defence to be clearly seen as belonging to the patient. It will not help if he accepts the patient's preferred view, namely that he has caused it. What is apparent, however, is that unless he learns to be adept in angry situations, he will probably find within himself a considerable reluctance to work to free himself from projections. He cannot work at this level if he sees his role as merely to please. A doctor who wishes to use and free himself from the power of projection must discover ways of being relaxed in disquieting situations. Unstructured, small-group experiences that enable study of interpersonal dynamics, similar to those sometimes referred to as 'Tavistock groups', are especially helpful for this (Shaffer and Galinsky, 1974), and the next chapter will consider anger in the consulting room.

When seeking to clarify a situation, people who stand outside it will often have a clarity about what is happening which those within it just cannot see. It is important therefore for the doctor to have someone to discuss his work with as he learns to handle projection, someone who will pay him the compliment of not pulling their punches, and will speak of what they believe is happening and explore it with him. This is probably essential when patients are not moving with their problems and when the doctor may well be colluding with them by projective identification, resulting in both of them being in a stuck state.

It is also useful to talk with other doctors in a group about their patient casework (Gosling *et al.*, 1967). The variety of different attitudes and understandings this can bring to bear on his work is especially helpful in reviewing his options and in perceiving the tell-tale clues to interlocking behaviours. It enables a doctor to clarify his own position and consider any aspects of his role which may be locking the patient into their problems. Colleagues can more easily spot the mind-sets that curtail and limit both him and the work he is doing. It is best for these groups to include a trained psychotherapist who can add grist to the group's mill in uncovering psychodynamic processes and the feelings engendered, and who will have had the training to handle these situations.

Doctors often find discussion of their work hard at first. After all, they very much put themselves into what they do, so it feels very personal. Also the work is about the private concerns of the patient and is undertaken behind closed doors. If discussion about work is seen as a social breaking of confidence, rather than as a legitimate and necessary part of any professional's work, a doctor may not consider it right to discuss what has gone on between him and his patient.

Difficulty in discussing work can be the result of wanting secret and fixed relationships with patients who are 'special' to the doctor, and where both patient and doctor are locked together in an un-helpful process. This dynamic is well described by Janet Mattinson (1979). She recounts her discovery of this difficulty, as having its seeds in the family in which the professionals were brought up and where the ability to have three-person relationships of any depth had not developed. If the relationship of the child with one of its parents did not allow sharing with the other parent, then secrecy and a 'special' relationship develop. This sort of relationship, while not really healthy or appropriate, can feel particularly exciting and intimate to the child, so that similar relationships may be sought in adult life. Doctors with this background may well not feel free to let a third person (a colleague) into the two-person, patient/doctor, 'special' relationship, through an open professional discussion about their work. Old childhood conflicts remain to be mirrored in later life, and here result in maintaining secrecy and in locking both doctor and patient into fixed childhood patterns of behaviour. There is stalemate with regard to the patient's 'dis-ease', and also with regard to the doctor's development of a more creative way of relating and working. There is stress for both of them that hides in the shared childhood longing to be exclusively and excitingly special – and there can be discomfort for the doctor's colleagues whose closer working relationship is spurned.

There is also the option of referring patients to a psychotherapist. In general, doctors seem to find this difficult (Woodhouse and Pengelly, 1991), and yet it is desirable and professional to pass a patient over to someone trained in a speciality, and to a level that few family doctors can attain. A doctor who is locked into projec-tions and finds it impossible to work his way free, could arguably be failing in his duty to the patient if he did not turn the patient over to a trained specialist. Woodhouse and Pengelly believe the difficulty lies in the anxieties of the medical profession and a defensive need for control.

There are other more general things a doctor can do to free himself from projective identification. It is important for him to have as varied and as full a life of his own as possible. Varied personal relationships enable him to have an intimate knowledge of the norms of being himself as he enters into the unhealthy relationships in which some patients will involve him. He will then more easily spot the different feel of the pathological inter-action, and so be more adroit in working to free himself from his part in any collusion. On top of these, a full, rich life will bring him satisfaction so that he needs his patients less for his own fulfilment.

Many doctors find that they are personally freer to be themselves – both in their work and out – through their own experience of psychotherapy or analysis. This experience helps a doctor to be aware of his own feelings. It helps him define his boundaries and know which feelings are his own, and therefore to know those that have come from other people. It enables him to be at home with feelings, to accept them, and through acceptance to become more fully aware. When personal psychotherapy is fully undertaken it is a remarkably freeing, exciting and fulfilling experience.

I hope these chapters have given an insight into the importance of projection for the family doctor. Its understanding is by no means a panacea, but undiscovered projections produce a consider-able psychological stress. Their discovery enables the doctor to understand people more readily and have more clarity about his work. It gives him a greater sense of his effectiveness, increases his job satisfaction and, as a result, improves his sense of well-being.

CHAPTER 11

Anger in the Consultation

In the early hours of the morning a doctor was called to a man with chest pain. He found that the patient was clearly having a heart attack and admitted him to hospital. Unfortunately the patient died the same night.

The following afternoon the doctor went to see the widow. The couple had moved to the area not long before so he had not known them well, but they had seemed friendly and he had not noticed anything especially unusual. Certainly he knew nothing that could have warned him of what was to come, other than that the husband had now died, of course.

He found that a daughter had come to be with her mother. It was quickly clear that they were going to give him a rough ride. They were both furious. He felt that they held him to be somehow responsible for what had happened and so he led them into recounting all that had taken place. It had seemed a long wait from the telephone call the wife had made that night to his arrival at the house, but she was also aware it had only been ten minutes. The ambulance had arrived quickly after he had called it. His treatment to relieve the chest pain with an intravenous injection had worked well, and the pain relief lasted until death. The hospital had given them immediate attention. There was nothing in all this that could rationally be considered to put the doctor at fault, and yet he clearly was being held responsible and was subject to a fury that hit him like a wall.

He was to learn a lot from this situation as he mulled it over later. Frequently doctors have to deal with death and, in so doing, can lose sight of the desolation it causes to those who were close and intricately involved in the dead person's life; but this reaction was out of all proportion to anything this experienced doctor had previously known, and was despite his having given them time and his considerate, aware response to their needs.

Subsequently the doctor learnt that on retirement the husband had persuaded his wife to move in order to be near a relative of his. She had not wished to move. They had gone through the whole stressful process of selling their house, buying another and moving in, only for the husband then to give up on life. She was left with a sense of the pointlessness of the move, and felt she would now have to reverse the whole process so as to return to the people she knew. She wished she had not let herself be steamrollered into moving by her husband and felt that the effort of the move had been too much for him and had caused his death. If only she had stood firm, she believed, he would still be alive; so she now felt responsible for his death and this guilt was very painful for her.

These feelings of guilt and badness, of loneliness and desolation are very common at death: they may be overpowering and difficult to carry. Anger at the dead partner for dying can mount to bursting point, and yet rationally this seems very unfair. The dead person did not want to die and the remaining relative may believe anger is not an acceptable feeling in the circumstances; so guilt for their anger is added to the huge burden of their strong, mixed feelings. Understandably, therefore, some people in these circumstances will deny their anger and project it elsewhere. Not surprisingly, doctors who are conveniently present at these times may be at the receiving end of anger and blame.

From the doctor's point of view this can be especially difficult. He has taken up medicine to try and alleviate distress and suffering. He may feel he has somehow let down those who die. He can easily be sucked into feeling he should have prevented the loved one's death and that therefore he has failed and caused the relatives' distress. Added to these feelings is the weight of his own emotions which inevitably occur in the presence of death, and which result from being with people who are shocked and facing the whole distressing process of loss and mourning.

People often have a perception that feeling angry is not professional (Bradbury, 1987) and certainly that showing it is quite out of order. In a doctor these attitudes will produce a dilemma, for, if he is to be himself, he must recognize his feelings and use them if he is to be effective.

Other people may go a long way to try and prevent anger in another, but attempts by a doctor to avoid 'making' patients angry may mean that he carries even more anger himself. Also in the last chapter it was observed that if a doctor is to challenge patient's projections he will need to be willing to face their anger on occasions. All in all, therefore, anger is a worthwhile area for analysis.

First there are several basic concepts which need stating so as to be able to build on them. Feelings are our own. It is *my* love I have for my wife, or *my* sadness at a parting. Few people would have any discomfort with these two examples. It is as if people are happy to own these feelings and lay claim to them, but often they do not feel at ease in claiming the feeling of anger. Frequently there are feelings of guilt about anger and people then judge themselves as not worthy because of it. Guilt and unworthiness will then underpin anger, causing further discomfort.

As with every feeling, all people experience anger. Human beings are subject to the whole range of human experience and angry feelings are included in the package. Anger is not bad in itself. Probably most people will agree with this and yet they may nonetheless behave as if they don't. It is as if people are able to agree with their intellect that there is no place for value judgements about anger, and yet they can behave as if this is not so.

And anger does not exclude other feelings. A man may love someone dearly and also feel anger in relation to them. Relationships hold a rich mix of feelings and no one of them can wipe out another. Also people can choose to prioritize their feelings, they can choose whether to express them or not, and usually they can choose how they will express them, when, how firmly and how obviously.

On the other hand, it really is useful if anger is expressed at a level appropriate to the situation at hand and if it is presented in a way judged likely to be receivable and useful to the other. 'I find I am feeling quite angry and am wondering why. Do you wish I had handled things differently at the meeting we've been discussing?' If it is spoken of in an honest open way, it enables discussion and increased understanding. There is no need for it to be manipulative, just observed and shared. It is then something that draws people closer together and is positive and creative.

What is often feared, however, is the pent-up venting of anger that comes from weeks – or even longer – of a whole series of angers that were not expressed at the time, and which can then burst out with a considerable head of steam. The force and uncontrolled nature of these outbursts can take even the angry person by surprise.

These experiences can be better understood if it is remembered how small children feel so single-mindedly and with their whole selves. I remember a little girl once saying to her friend, 'I *hate* you'. She really shouted it out and looked as if she really did hate her friend. Her whole body and personality seemed to be involved in that vibrant statement. Perhaps it is as a result of the child's total involvement in a feeling that later, as adults, people can believe anger cannot exist alongside other feelings, and they see anger as all consuming or even as dangerous. A child's understanding of murder must surely be that one person was phenomenally angry with another. The child cannot comprehend psychosis, nor the fact that healthy adults may have grades of anger and are able to choose to act on it or not. The fear of the 'all or nothing' perception of the child can live on in the adult if it is not thought out.

But what happens when anger is legitimately expressed? As an example I will take the rather trivial situation of a friend having trodden on my toe. I feel angry. Anger exists in me: it is experienced and owned. There may then be a checking out. 'Are you all right? You seem rather clumsy. That really hurt my toe.' Depending on why my friend says he trod on my toe, I might then respond with, 'I did not find your prank funny.'

It is noteworthy that in this example I could choose to have found the episode a joke. So there is an element of choice in me when I focus on anger and it temporarily predominates over other feelings. This choice is something that people can develop largely through acceptance of their feelings. For instance, I might choose both to treat the episode as a joke and to express annoyance at my friend's readiness to inflict pain. The feeling of anger is mine to use as I choose, just because it is my feeling.

Similarly, a doctor can say to a patient: 'It makes it difficult to look after you when you often fail to turn up for appointments, and this time you have arrived an hour late without any apparent concern. I find it hard to settle down to the consultation in these circumstances.' That is a gentle, though firm, statement. The doctor owns his frustration and outlines its effects on their relationship and work. Of course patients, too, need to be given respect for all their feelings, and these can be quite strong when the doctor is running late. The feelings engendered can usefully be verbalized: 'I'm sorry I'm running late. It must be annoying to have had to wait so long.'

All feelings can be used as a defence, and anger is no exception. If there is a distressing feeling, for example of vulnerability, or the fear of loss, then a person may unconsciously attempt to drown it with anger. This way they disguise their vulnerability. The underlying tender feelings are overlain with anger and their vulnerability goes unacknowledged and camouflaged, even from themselves. The anger, meanwhile, can be out of all proportion to its apparent cause.

A man rang his family practitioner and exploded with annoyance at the receptionist, saying that the practice had not been in touch with him after he had been seen in the hospital Out Patients three days before. The receptionist was confused and indignant. When the doctor later sat down with the patient it became clear that he was distressed by a provisional diagnosis of probable cancer and he could hardly cope with his fear, nor with his feeling that life might well be over before he had achieved what he wanted. It transpired that the man's wife had left him the previous year and their two children blamed him for this. He had not yet been able to work

111

through to a more realistic relationship with his teenage children, and now all hope of doing so seemed suddenly to have been torn away. His sense of hopelessness, and an expectation of an imminent and lonely end, were too great. Unable to cope with these feelings, he made contact with people by covering up his vulnerability with anger which he directed at anything that came readily to hand. He covered over one strong but painful set of emotions with another strong emotion which was acceptable to him. His more vulnerable feelings of confusion, indignation and other distresses were projected and had been picked up by the receptionist.

Initially, however, both the receptionist and the doctor tended to assume the practice had done something to deserve the anger. Only when the doctor faced the man's anger did he develop a contact with the man's real concerns that enabled both doctor and patient to be in touch with the realities. The doctor could not have done this unless he had been willing to share something of the hopelessness and despair that so distressed the patient. The man was not only using anger to cover up his distress, but also to displace his feelings at the unfairness of life – perhaps from his wife and children – onto the practice. There was a cry for help in his behaviour – so many things were happening, all interweaving.

This example is given as an illustration of anger being used to cover over and swamp an overpoweringly distressful mix of vulnerable, tender feelings. Facing the anger enabled the doctor to be relieved of the assumption of its personal nature and so not be drawn into identifying with the projector. It left him, and subsequently the receptionist (for something of this needed to be discussed with her), both able to free themselves from a sense of having been at fault in some way.

Using anger as a defence is like unconsciously choosing to give angry feelings a priority and precedence over the more tender, painful feelings which an individual may unconsciously wish to defend himself against. Doctors meet many frightened and worried people and in these circumstances many of them defend in this way. It is therefore a frequent experience.

The use of anger as a defence occurs in people who are able to express anger. What, though, of those who have difficulty doing so, the people who have a perception (developed and absorbed through their upbringing) that angry feelings are not acceptable, that they are bad or dangerous? Any sense of anger would then result in guilt and these painful and potent feelings are often then defended against in one way or another. In these people, far from using anger as a defence, they defend themselves from it. The possible defence mechanisms can be summarized and listed as:

blaming others, displacing the anger so that it is expressed to someone else less valued or feared, denial of the feeling so that it is not recognized and, finally, by projection into someone else, either in the present or across time. There may be a combination of these defences, but first I want to briefly look at each in turn.

People can distance themselves from their anger by considering it was caused by someone else. Rather than accept that they are angry, they blame someone else for making them angry and as a result can feel far less responsible for it: 'You have made me angry.' This type of attitude was well portrayed in the Laurel and Hardy films 'Look what you made me do.' Clearly the attitude is that they cannot help but be angry because of what someone else has done. Someone else is to blame. However, while blaming others in an attempt to ease their guilt, they, by implication, maintain that others are responsible for their feelings; it suggests that other people have control over their responses, as if they themselves are puppets.

Another strategy of defence is displacement. We are used to seeing someone in a comedy who, for instance, feeling angry at what he has just heard, turns away to kick the dog; or a man who, rather than be angry at what he has heard about his wife, displaces it by taking it out on the bearer of the news. It is easy to imagine this latter man's predicament as he feels his anger and yet is aware of how much he and his wife love each other. The bearer of the news may be unknown to him and will not be seen again. No doubt for him there was less anxiety about his guilt if the messenger was made the focus for his anger. In these examples the angry person is both blaming others for his feelings and displacing punishment onto a different person or object.

Similarly, in a medical situation, there is the example given at the beginning of this chapter, of the recently widowed woman who displaced her anger onto the first person that came along – her new doctor – even though he could in no way have been responsible for her husband's death and, indeed, had efficiently and effectively come to their aid. There are many occasions when the doctor receives displaced anger.

Denial of a feeling is another defence that is an unconscious attempt to clear that individual of his unwanted feelings. If guilt and shame about anger are great, it can be eased if the anger is totally denied. The angered person may say: 'I have no anger. I am never angry. I'm not that sort of person.' On the surface these people may seem easy to be with. Yet, at a different level, and given time with them, they are very difficult to be with. They do not speak their minds, but their aggression slides out sideways, quickly and quietly as if in disguise. They have been described as 'passive-aggressive personalities'.

People's denial of anger may, however, go a step further so that the denied anger is projected onto another person. The angry person has, unconsciously, totally denied the feeling and is not aware of it, but it will inevitably have its own life and it is dumped on to someone else who can find himself feeling angry without being sure why.

To be on the receiving end of this process can be an extremely powerful experience. I remember once being at a meeting with a small group of people. There was a man there whom I did not know. He was very tense and ill at ease with himself and seemed to spar tangentially with everyone and anyone. In the short hour or so of that meeting he bickered with one person after another, although it was never clear why. It was all done as if by sleight of hand, with a fixed smile and gentle voice, and only after later consideration did I realize much of what I am now describing.

The meeting finished and, talking to one or two of the members of the group, I checked out my perception of his aggressiveness and received some confirmation. On my way home I became aware of how uncomfortable I was. I was angry, my heart was beating fast, I was breathing deeper and faster than I physically needed, I felt anxious, disagreeable, ill at ease and almost physically ill. My feelings had the quality of ones that were not my own. I soon felt exhausted and this unsettled state persisted in me right up to my eventually getting off to sleep that night. It was extremely unpleasant. I could not put my mind to anything of any consequence for the remains of the evening, nor, not knowing what the anger was about, could I at the time understand myself. Such was the power of this man's projected anger.

There was a further aspect to this group situation. After the meeting, and when I had arrived home, I found myself thinking, 'I need a drink'. In retrospect I found this disconcerting as I was not having a drink for pleasure but to 'drown' feelings that I could do little with. I have noticed this on other occasions. 'Needing a drink' can alert me to the probability of projected feeling.

This experience of projected anger brings to mind how I sometimes have felt after a surgery with particularly angular and difficult patients. Accumulative projections from various patients, one after another, can have an exhausting effect and leave me feeling rotten – as if I am rotten. I feel annoyance and have a sense of being blameworthy.

People who project feelings sometimes proceed a stage further and blame the recipient for the very feelings they have themselves projected onto them. For instance, Mr X, having projected his anger onto Mr Y, may then make the observation that Mr Y is angry: 'Mr Y is angry and of course I am not like that. I do not like anger.' So Mr Y is criticized for carrying Mr X's anger, adding insult to injury. Mr X can feel self-righteous and comfortable, while Mr Y is left really fuming.

A doctor may sometimes need to spend time after a surgery reflecting on his feelings, so as to remain firm in his self-perception and to counter a succession of patients' mixed bags of disquieting, angry, projected feelings. Otherwise he may not understand where these feelings are from, what they are about, what peg to hang them on, and find it almost impossible to do anything with them. They seem to have no cause and therefore often have a 'bursting out of control' quality, and can disruptively hang around in him for a long time.

Accurately perceiving the projected feeling's source also gives insight into the patient's inner world. People who project their anger cannot express what frustrates them, so that their effectiveness suffers and they themselves suffer in silent impotence.

By working at it, the doctor can learn to recognize the quality of feelings that are not his own. Such focused sensitivity enables him to use, or alternatively diminish, his internal acceptance of projected feelings. By developing this ability he frees himself both from believing the feelings are his own, and also from a resulting perception of himself as being chaotic and irrational. As a result, he can be far more comfortable when working with a projecting patient. Similarly, by helping patients to understand and acknowledge what is going on in them, they, too, move towards being more satisfyingly themselves.

So far, projection of anger has been described as occurring in the present and towards someone who is conveniently there at the time, but there is another possibility which occurs when a projection also involves a transfer of feeling across time.

Recently I heard of the way one of the High Street banks had behaved in what was, to my mind, a crushingly bad way to someone whose business was secured with a bank loan. He had business orders for many months to come but had customers who were slow in paying him, causing him difficulty with cash flow. Almost without warning the bank foreclosed on the loan, forcing my friend close to bankruptcy, and then obtained knowledge of his private account held at another branch, to turn the screws even more.

Now the rights and wrongs of this are not the point of bringing this example. I felt angry at what I heard. Part of this anger was my own, and part my friend's. I did nothing with the anger – for

115

instance I did not ask to talk to the bank manager about it on my friend's behalf (which anyway would have been quite inappropriate). However, a week or two later and when visiting my own, different, High Street bank, I found myself angrily reacting to some minor procedural slip of no real consequence and certainly not anything I would normally be inconvenienced or annoyed about. Here was anger at something in the recent past coming out in the present. I was transferring the feeling across time as well as onto an inappropriate person. Only in retrospect did I become conscious of the process.

Such 'transference' (Freud, 1915) of feeling can be extremely powerful, and especially so when the original event was a half forgotten and seemingly unrelated situation that had occurred long before. For example, as a child a patient had often found himself entering his father's study only to be belittled and made to feel ineffective and inconsequential. Years later, and as an adult, this same person enters another authority figure's room (that of a doctor) and this unconsciously throws him back to the relationship with his father, and his strong and previously unexpressed feelings now come flooding back. The original situation and the person associated with this sudden upsurge of feeling lie in his forgotten past. The present situation is distorted by past feelings, transferred to the present.

All sorts of other complicating dynamics can be added to this scenario. The patient is surprised by these feelings, is confused, and may perhaps consider it must be the doctor that has caused his anger, and blames him for them. (Indeed, the doctor has unknowingly reminded him of his past and has triggered his feelings, although he has not caused them.) The patient may then give the doctor a sense of being responsible and bad, and the doctor can find himself vulnerably accepting the patient's projection and, as a result, try to placate him by doing far more for him than is necessary or useful.

This is an example of a shift of feelings to an inappropriate person across a great deal of time; from the distant and only partially understood childhood past, to the present. Because the past is forgotten and the process is unseen, it lends the present feeling great strength through being an unconscious force. This 'transference' of feeling can alter a person's perception of the reality of the here and now out of all recognition. Present reality becomes lost in a mix of ungrounded, past feelings.

All the defensive mechanisms described here can interweave, one following another, and make a most complex structure that people lock into, and which tie and restrict them from being themselves

116

and from acting in their own, or each other's, best interests. They take up emotional energy and are exhausting and stressful.

To end this chapter, here is an example from a colleague's practice of just such a mix. An elderly woman presented herself at the reception desk and demanded to see my colleague straight away. She said she was going to sue the practice and wanted to talk to him. She was personally offensive and pushy with the receptionist. Here was anger that seemed to be displaced onto the receptionist.

My colleague felt angry as he heard this, and when he saw the patient he found that this feeling increased. She told him that her grandson Tim was in hospital with leukaemia, and that his partners had not made the diagnosis fast enough. My friend checked the boy's notes and the reality was that Tim had been seen once with a common cold, and again a week later because a haemorrhagic rash had developed. A blood test, and his admission to hospital, followed that same day. In truth, appropriate speedy action had been taken and the diagnosis had been made as quickly as possible. Here was displaced and projected anger along with defensive blaming, but my friend did not yet know more. He needed to focus on Grandma who was doing the projecting, rather than the boy.

He sat back and verbally observed that it must all be very difficult for her. It transpired that she was now looking after the other two grandchildren so that her daughter could stay at the hospital with Tim.

Grandma was distressed for Tim, distressed for her daughter, and distressed for herself and her husband. It became clear that one source of her anger resulted from feeling trapped, in that her elderly husband found it especially stressful having the two fit and energetic grandchildren in the house all the time, and was having to take far more of his angina tablets as a result. She felt that she had no option but to take care of the grandchildren but, because of her husband's angina, the children's presence might cause her to lose him. The quiet, relaxed, contented retirement they had been having and enjoying together had suddenly blown up in their faces. Her fear at her threatened loss was too great. Life was unfair. Unconsciously she looked for someone to blame and then anger could displace her anxiety. Someone should take this stress away, she felt, and apportioning blame makes disease and death seem not to be an inevitable part of life. In the process of blaming, she also displaced her anger onto my friend's colleagues and staff. He, however, had faced the anger, looked into the reality of the situation and freed himself from feeling the practice was responsible. He had then looked into why she was angry and got

117

her to talk about it. Her admission of frustration, and then owning her own distress and vulnerability, began to free the doctor from her projected confusion and anger.

The doctor arranged to see the grandmother again. He was to learn that, years ago when she was in her teens, her father had had some ongoing debilitating illness. Her mother had been the only breadwinner and so this woman's teens were filled with the adult chores of housework and nursing her father. She was the one who used to contact the doctor and he would make comments about how important she was to the household and how dependent they were on her. No doubt he had intended to encourage her but, unwittingly, he had increased her sense of entrapment. As a result of all this she had lost a much-loved boyfriend who had tired of waiting in the wings as she toiled on her parents' behalf. She had had a very busy life since, she said, and sometimes wondered what it would have been like with the first boyfriend. She believed it would have been easier as she knew he had entered a profession.

Just as, in the distant past, she had lost her boyfriend through nursing her father, now, in the present, she feared she might also lose her husband through another's illness. Life had opened out in their old age and she and her husband had been enjoying each other's company. Was this experience to be lost to her yet again?

What had particularly seemed to drive this home to her had been her feelings as she queued at the reception desk at the doctor's surgery. This, she later realized, had suddenly made her feel she was wasting her time, and she felt totally trapped and angry. It reminded her of those teenage years when she had been responsible for her father. She felt once more that the doctors would expect her to act 'responsibly' and look after her daughter's needs, rather than relieve her from them as she desired, and this compounded her feeling of being trapped. Her anger had immediately mounted in a way that surprised her.

Here was the process of feelings transferred across time from her early life to the present day; transferred from a person in the past to someone in the present; and all brought on by her recurring feeling of entrapment. This complex matrix and burden of feeling was difficult for her to carry or unravel. Her usual channel for sharing a burden through talking was denied to her by her wish to protect her husband because of his life-threatening angina, and she dumped the feelings onto my colleague's staff and partners.

Blaming, displacing, projecting and transference are all ways in which people may shift responsibility for their feelings from themselves, and often result in a trap for the unwary – and perhaps over-caring – doctor.

CHAPTER 12

Doctors' Attitudes to Patients

In earlier chapters, a doctor's attitudes were explored in relation to both himself and to his role. It is now time to consider his attitudes to patients. Two things have emerged in the book so far that make this chapter important. First, a large element of stress develops out of a doctor's own attitudes; secondly, his attitudes and assumptions may result in projections onto a patient which will lock the two into an inflexible and stressful system.

I remember a family doctor saying that he felt like a fly in a spider's web, one of those flies that at first glance look glistening and fat but, on closer inspection, are seen to have been sucked dry and are empty shells with no life juices left. He was, he said, afraid that the draft of air as the next patient came in through the consulting room door would cause him to disintegrate into a little shower of dust, and even this was in danger of being quickly blown away. I knew something of what he described. Self-preservation is essential for doctors. They must maintain the will, ability and time to move into the sunlight and find their own revitalizing warmth.

These exhausted feelings are increased when the doctor's role is being idealized, not so much by patients, but rather by the doctor's own idealizations. Often a doctor's parents will have encouraged him to take up a career in medicine when he was young, and while this may be for a whole variety of reasons, their attitudes will frequently have been picked up by their child. If, for instance, they have recommended medicine because they see doctoring as a really worthwhile profession that represents the height of caring, the doctor's resulting idealization of medical work may reveal itself through such phrases as 'the best' or 'first class' care.

Idealized concepts of work cannot possibly be fulfilled and must therefore result in a sense of failure. The unattainable is inevitably surrounded by feelings of inadequacy and guilt, with a consequent loss of self-esteem. But these disturbing feelings can be so defended against that a doctor will press himself into doing more and more in an attempt to relieve himself of them, and often he will do so to a degree that is no longer appropriate and not even helpful to his patients. Doctors therefore must think through what is appropriate to the task and situation at hand,

and aim for what is likely to be effective for the patient's problems, rather than merely to maintain some ideal.

A common idealization is that patients must be pleased and the doctor must be seen to be 'nice', and yet, of course, the doctor's prime task is to be efficient and effective. With these objectives he may frequently need to jeopardize a patient's short-term pleasure as, ultimately, being effective is the only real way to please a patient. The doctor's skills must therefore frequently include ways of *not* giving patients what they want. Sometimes, for instance, he will need to educate them to a wider need and point the way to its fulfilment. If this process is to be effective, the doctor will need to find ways of considerately expressing his inner, more challenging feelings, such as his anger, and he will not always be able to wrap up what a patient may find uncomfortable in an immediately acceptable way.

There is another common idealization that frequently results in a doctor feeling himself to be responsible for patients. It is as if he sees himself as powerful and the patient as dependent on him. It is a perception that may often find a comfortable fit between male doctors and female patients, or between the adult doctor and a teenager, but it is common enough with patients of all types and is particularly powerful because of the authority the doctor holds as a result of his medical knowledge. This undoubted area of authority is allowed to spill out into other areas where it has no right to be – for instance, into assuming value judgements for a patient's personal decisions. For a patient it can be comforting to assume his doctor has increased (although unreal) powers so that they can relinquish their own responsibility, but for the doctor it presupposes that he is more able and powerful than the patient in arranging their lives, and that is presumptuous to say the least.

It seems to be a variation of this attitude that is reflected in doctors who say that, whatever a doctor does, he must not take away a patient's hope, or, alternatively, that the doctor must 'give patients hope'. This is voiced fairly frequently and usually by hospital doctors in discussions about how much should be said to patients in relation to their fatal illness. When those saying this are questioned, their belief seems to have arisen out of an attitude that the patient should be protected. The patient is treated as if he were unable to face the realities of life with all the full breadth of feeling that life rightly holds, and at the same time there is the assumption that the doctor is not only able to face these things but should do so for the patient. To clarify, let me say that I am sure the way bad news is given is an art in itself, but protecting the patient is unnecessarily stressful for both the people concerned: the patient is held back from self-understanding and from being as fully responsible for his life as possible, while the doctor busies himself with someone else's responsibilities, confusing them with his own. Meanwhile, their relationship is weakened by an authoritarian, belittling attitude, and sometimes by falsity.

It may be helpful to briefly explore a possible origin of the human need to take responsibility for others. Recently my wife and I were camping in France on the sort of site where it is easy to observe the other families camped around. A few had small babies with them, and I was struck once again by the care parents will give to their little baby. They take complete responsibility. Mothers especially seem to know just what is required and are usually easy and relaxed about it. Some fathers are not so in tune with an infant's needs, and yet most of them clearly have that same sense of responsibility.

On the campsites there were, of course, families with older children. Some were not so relaxed and it seemed to me that in these families the parents were maintaining their sense of responsibility long past their child's need for total care. These children were not free to follow their own interests or do their own thing without considerable parental anxiety and a degree of control quite inappropriate to their age. It seemed that these parents had not adjusted to changed circumstances, their childrens' increased ages and the greater safety on the campsite. They had not let go of a type of responsibility that was no longer appropriate.

All humans have experienced someone else's care when they were children and, no doubt, some part of every adult will look back with a sense of longing to the time when they did not have to take on adult responsibility for themselves, and they mourn the loss of the age of innocence. Nevertheless, child care is not a relevant care for adults, and if appropriate adult care is not thought through, it can be assumed that 'care' means a return to elements of the protectiveness and reduced responsibility rightly extended to a child. I see this process of letting go of one type of responsibility and developing another, pertinent to doctors as they consider their attitudes to patients. Each situation, let alone each person, will require thoughtful consideration.

For a doctor to hold responsibility may sound demanding and even restrictive, but there is a laid-back responsibility that is not compelling, or manipulative; it is a non-pressuring, background 'fact'. It is a condition of being 'response-able'. Being able to respond (though not necessarily doing so), must entail being able to see the crux of a situation so that the insight alone is what is available to others, leaving them to be active in their own lives. The doctor does well to define the responsibility of his various roles: with the sick, the incapacitated and disabled, with the patient's family, with the man who is temporarily down, with the patient who will never be anything else but down perhaps because of a permanent personality disorder, and with his own role as doctor within and for society. He must free himself from his internal pressures which engage him in unnecessary and, in the longer term, unhelpful activity, saving his energy for his own necessary endeavours.

And not accepting an active responsibility for the patient is especially relevant when, progressively, members of society claim in the courts that their doctor has made a wrong decision about their treatment. It is important that the patient be given his options and that the doctor then carries out the patient's chosen treatment. This does not remove the doctor's responsibility for whatever he physically undertakes to do on their behalf, but makes for a necessarily different background atmosphere.

If the patient is to be response-able for himself, then the responsible thing for the response-able doctor to do, is to encourage, enable and challenge the patient to develop the condition of being response-able for themselves.

I am reminded of a paper, whose reference detail I cannot for the life of me now recall, in which the researchers were trying to uncover what might be peculiar to families who were judged to be especially effective in their lives and in living together. They selected two groups of families: one that they considered (by carefully drawn criteria) to be dysfunctional, and another group who functioned well. They then videoed them on a day-to-day basis with cameras mounted in the rooms of their homes. They could then peruse these recordings at their leisure.

This careful and thorough work resulted in their postulating that effective families seem to have a readiness and ability to discuss and examine how they have interacted when they are at sixes and sevens with each other and so clarify how they had become disrupted. After developing a clear understanding of each other and of their interaction, they then get on with life. They do not indulge in this work of self-understanding all the time, but are easily able to do so when they have become dysfunctional. This example gives a cameo of being response-able within relationships. It is as if being responsible for oneself enables the individual to interrelate, as if each is defined as a person and, in the process, become clearly available to relate as the full person they are. They do not, for example, get drawn into the half relationship that results from attempts to protect another person. They deal, and leave others to deal, with realities. There is then no interweaving of projection and projective identification that depersonalizes.

At times there will be conflict between the patients' understanding of their need or wish and the doctor's way of working from his understanding of his role as free from projective identification. These conflicts are inevitable, and will produce creative tension. They can be explored to advantage and, while the doctor may believe it appropriate and choose to accompany a patient during a time of particular struggle, in the end he must also withdraw and return to a position of being response-able.

There is a further complicating factor for doctors with regard to responsibility. With physical illness the doctor's diagnosis is often followed by an ongoing responsibility to treat the patient's condition. His medical knowledge brings a responsibility to prescribe and monitor the patient's progress; thus, in physical illness he will often be active on the patient's behalf. In the psychological area of a doctor's work things are different. The relationship between patient and doctor is close while the two engage in puzzling over the patient's problems and they both focus on intimate areas of the patient's life, but when a psychological diagnosis is defined and the options open to the patient have been signposted, the intimacy must end. The doctor's responsibility and activity on the patient's behalf must rightly finish. It demands he hand over any responsibility he has taken in their lives and that he walk away as cleanly as possible, and certainly free of tarnishing falsity.

This movement out of intimacy may result in a sense of loss in both patient and doctor which can sometimes cause a doctor to hang on by claiming a continuing role. However, the patient is now responsible for using the insights he has gained, if that is his wish, and in doing so he will both discover and use his own strength and power by taking responsibility for his life. An example of the process would be of the doctor labelling the patient as being overly 'anxious' and leaving him to do something about it. It is the patient who must make the decisions, such as to ring a psychotherapist and start work on the diagnosed anxiety. The patient may need to return to the doctor, but only to have the diagnosis reiterated or to be firmly reminded of the need for that self-referral. Because the doctor does not hold responsibility, there is no place for him to have a sinking feeling as he again sees the patient's notes on his pile at the start of a surgery. Nor is the doctor locking himself into seeing that patient every first Monday in the month to do – he knows not what.

There is in this a sense of there being boundaries to each of the two involved, of responsible areas defined and the patient and doctor each in charge of his own self. The doctor's own freedom enables him to view his patients with genuine friendliness and regard. His behaviour shows that personal freedom is possible and that will challenge the patient to grasp it too.

However, some people hold an idealized view that a good relationship is one in which there is such an understanding in each of the other that nothing needs to be said. It would seem to be like the early relationship of a mother with her infant when care must be total; the baby cannot sort anything out for itself, and the mother seems attuned to its every whim, even though nothing has been said. That is a suitable relationship for mother and infant, but something quite different is appropriate between adults. Adults do discover their own detailed wishes and differences; they are able to live more exciting exploratory lives; and they can verbally negotiate mutually satisfactory, yet different, stances. Adults need to be separate from parents, from their children, spouse and friends, and their individual boundaries must be constantly redefined. For instance, in a growing family, boundaries will be different for the father in his role with an eight-year-old son, from those with a fourteen-year-old daughter, and they will change as both son and daughter get older and marry. They will further change when he is old and his son and daughter support him in his failing health, so the changes in a father's role are not only to do with the growing personalities of the children, but also the development of the father as he continues to mature and age. Boundaries must continuously be adjusted. They can be moved so as to include what the individual perceives and wishes himself to be, or to exclude what he chooses not to be. It requires the hard work of clarifying perceptions and redefining those made in the past which now need replacing with more adult or up-to-date realities. It is not a forcing into a mould, but rather an observational activity that includes discovery of feelings, thoughts and actions, along with the weighing-up of values, concerns and desires.

And as with the individual, so the doctor must define the boundaries between himself and his role as doctor. It is complicated, and his own life changes will mean that their consideration and adjustment will be an ongoing challenge but, while it requires hard thinking, it also enables the doctor to be finer tuned to his varying tasks and to function more freely as a person. Any lack of definition may result either in a doctor moving out into the patient's area of responsibility or a too-isolated doctor becoming even more separate so that he is not free to engage with patients at an effective level. A doctor's clarity about his role and his work of self-definition will free him to be flexible. He will serve as a model of freedom which his patients find enacted in the relationship on offer, and which in turn gives the patient permission, and a better chance, to discover what personal boundaries can do for him.

One doctor planning to enter general practice told me: 'Family practice is an interesting job in itself, but there really is icing on the cake if only we can see people as individuals and make contact with them as the human beings they are rather than just as patients.' He went on to expand this in relation to colleagues and staff in the practice and was, I think, also telling of life experience in general. It is an observation that is deceptive in its apparent simplicity. I wonder what it is that the doctor defends against by seeing individual people all clumped together in a pigeon-hole labelled 'patients'. If such defensive compartmentalization results in the loss of the icing on the cake, it must be because of some considerable gain. Let us try to tease out what this may be.

The following experience can help to elucidate these defences. When I first came to this quite widely spread, rural practice, my wife and I set up home outside the practice area because houses for sale were few and far between. Then once our sons were settled in the village school we did not want to uproot them again when more suitably placed houses came onto the market, so we stayed where we were. We have not, therefore, found ourselves getting to know many patients socially. However, it so happened that there were two patients I did particularly get to know. One had my sons round to his farm to ferret and, as I was involved as 'chauffeur', I sometimes joined in. This man also had the hobby of fly-fishing and taught me its skills, drawing me into the fraternity of those enthralled by the tug of a fish on a line.

The other patient I knew particularly well had had wide experience of world travel. His resulting ability to stand back and observe, along with an exceptionally open nature, attracted me to him, and I would drop in for an occasional cup of tea and a break before late afternoon surgery.

Now it so happened that one weekend, when I was off duty, both these men died. To be told this on Monday morning was a distressing experience. I did not have much energy to work: I needed to lick my wounds and be alone.

I suspect this experience is relevant in explaining why doctors may defensively and firmly categorize as 'patients' those they work amongst. Kept in that role, the doctor can allow that these people, however likeable, are at least potentially ill and liable to both suffering and death. Patients die, but doctors and their friends must be held to be different. Keep, then, the category of 'patients' quite separate from 'doctors', to define those who suffer and die – and the doctor can better face his work. This is, however, to hold an attitude that disease and dying are exclusively relevant to patients, a form of projection. But the icing of reality excludes projections.

The reality of all relationships is that they engage feelings and yet there is a common belief or attitude in medical training that a doctor's feelings should not be involved. However, doctors need to admit their feelings towards patients. For instance, they no doubt like to have good feelings towards people – it helps a self-image of their being nice people – but they need to admit the dislikes and stronger feelings they have for aspects of patients. Unless they admit these feelings they can find themselves unconsciously covering them up with 'proof' of concern, by being good, caring, totally giving (but exhausted) doctors.

Without doubt, feelings can be strong between patient and doctor; both attractive and unattractive feelings. They bring richness and depth to the work that they do together. But it is the doctor's definition of himself and his clarity about his own and the patient's roles, as well as his own and his patient's feelings, that frees the two in their intimacy. There is some definable relationship, other than rigidly compartmentalized categories of 'friend' (with feeling), or 'patient' (with no feeling), which allows a richness of relating between doctor and patient and still enables a doctor to be a professional, freed from over-involvement. Such a position enables an effective carer rightly to preserve his deepest involvement and vulnerabilities for his family and personal friends, and at the same time enables a greater relevant sensitivity at work. Every doctor must seek this for himself.

There are, of course, other difficulties which may arise if a doctor fails to keep people who are patients in a different relationship to that of close friends. There can be confusion when patients are very open. It can feel very seductive and this may seem even more so when their medical condition requires that they submit to intimate handling of their bodies. But a patient's openness is a direct result of the problems he has come about. That is his motivation in seeking the doctor's company, and the resulting, and relevant, relationship is not to be mistaken for a full one. There is clearly a whole range of sexual feelings that are safe only within firm medical boundaries; the patient's need is merely for a working relationship – difficult enough in itself. Doctors do well to maintain an involved, full life outside work, not only for their own richness of life, but also to help them maintain their involved, yet limited, role. Life for the doctor, as measured by time, may mostly be taken up by work, but the greatest quality of intimacy needs to be maintained at home. The doctor's interest and warm feelings will sometimes feel dangerously close to spilling over, but his actions are within his own control.

I believe it is important, when defining relationships with patients, to hold onto the fact that the relationship exists to facilitate the patients' work on themselves. That is why they have come to him and that is the contractual focus for the doctor's involvement. He may get a sense of satisfaction from his work, but otherwise the relationship is for the patient. It is a one-way relationship, quite unlike the relationship with friends which will rightly be a two-way involvement. A fuller emotional commitment is not appropriate, nor compatible to a doctor's task.

Perhaps, though, it is this perception of working for other people's good that so often results in doctors being placed on a pedestal. Doctors are more aware these days of patients idealizing them in this way. They sometimes comment and laugh about it, but frequently they rather like it and take it for granted. There are, for instance, the patients who show deference and are 'good' patients or, perhaps, when the doctor takes his car to the garage, he may be given some preference. 'Why not?' the doctor may ask, 'After all, it is they who are putting me on a pedestal', or 'It helps make up for the unpleasant aspects of being a doctor.' And yet patients who put the doctor on a pedestal must inevitably have some reason. It may be, for example, to keep themselves, by comparison, in the gutter – such is their lack of self-esteem. For others it may be in the unconscious belief that if the doctor is held to be a god, they feel secure that he will be able to keep them alive. But whatever the reason, this unrealistic attitude towards their doctor does not in the end help the patient's development. Nor could the doctor be put on a pedestal unless his stance was of extraordinarily inhibited passivity. The top of a pedestal is small and restricts movement; its height prevents good contact with those on the ground and causes sustained isolation. It is therefore something a doctor chooses for himself, but which restricts his humanity and reduces his effectiveness. I believe he fulfils his role best by working from a position alongside the patient. He needs to be neither above nor below; not dragging behind, nor pulling from in front; but rather standing alongside, accurately informing them of his observations.

There may be a belief that the doctor has to take control for the patient. It is my experience that some of the most uncomfortable people to be with are those whose need for control spills out into control of those around them. With them I feel constrained, stifled and ignored as a person. I do not believe that anyone, in the long run, really enjoys these relationships. Similarly, control of

127

a patient by a doctor is uncomfortable and inhibiting. It is better if the doctor learns to adjust. Some very anxious patients calm down only when control is exercised but, with time, their way forward is to learn to take charge of themselves.

Some doctors will not wish to explore the various possible psychological avenues of their role but, for those who do, fixed preconceived ideas of how a doctor must behave will make for reduced flexibility. For instance, some patients are unable to be open and may require the doctor to reach out to them. They may be locked into themselves like mice, hardly daring to peep out of their holes at life and unable to risk making contact with others. In this situation there can be a psychologically seductive quality to the doctor's role. What I find I have done occasionally over the years is to offer myself as bait: 'Come out and join me.' More than that, to a degree, I have gently moved in alongside the patient and, having established some sense of safety for them, I have then enticed them out to join in with the human race. In turn the patient's intense loneliness and isolation may also have an unconscious, psychologically seductive quality to it that may draw from the doctor an attempt to save them from their loneliness by, as it were, staying with them rather than only accompanying them briefly as they leave their isolated seclusion. In these situations it helps in adjusting to the psychological intimacy for the doctor to be clear that it is a quite separate situation from social intimacy. It is as if the doctor, if he is able to adjust to the variety of situations he finds in patients, can use himself in many different ways once he clears himself of preconceived ideals and set ideas of how he 'should' work.

That a doctor will probably respond to something about the individual patient with increased interest is, of course, natural enough. Educationalists say that a child will do well at school if he can draw the teacher's interest, and that it is the child who does not have this magnetism or ability and whom the teacher may therefore find uninteresting who languishes alone in his difficulties and, as a result, does not do well. For a doctor the situation is different in that he is normally dealing with one person at a time, but there is a need for him to offer time and effort according to a patient's need and despite any personal discomfort. For example, in a patient who is depressed, it may be useful for the doctor to conceptualize his role as requiring him to hold in his mind's eye that person's potential for a full life, rather than respond only to how he experiences the patient.

It may at first seem strange to say it, but the doctor must also learn to let people go. There is a need to come close to a patient, but there is also the need to expect that the patient will, in the end, move out of the relationship with the doctor and start to use his new-found skills and experience in developing full relationships outside the consulting room; that he will turn acquaintances into friends; allow friends to become intimates; and then to let an intimate into that most vulnerable relationship of all, that of an ongoing partner. The doctor must stand back from his work with the patient and focus on the patient's longer-term need. He must allow the ending, learn to accept the sadness of parting and find real, though brief, encounters with people exciting enough. As Cecil Day Lewis put it in a poem dedicated to Sean, who I suspect was his son:

> ... selfhood begins with a walking away,
> And love is proved in the letting go.
> (C. Day Lewis, 1977)

If a doctor can allow himself to examine his attitudes to his patients then there are many subtle adjustments that can enhance his effectiveness and, incidentally, relieve his burden. For instance, Enid Balint and her co-authors, in *Six Minutes for the Patient* (1973), describe the scenario of work with patients done briefly and intermittently down the years. It can be very sustaining and helpful. The patient is periodically 'held' safely, enabling him to feel safe enough to make changes to his life while not excessively burdening the doctor. But it is a way of working that depends on the attitude that it is the patient who does the work of adjusting, the doctor only being there to help him to focus and feel safe enough for his task. It presumes that the patient is responsible for his work which therefore can, and will, be pursued between visits to the doctor. If the doctor holds this attitude for the patient, then all that many people require is to see the doctor when their adaptation process becomes stuck.

Dame Cecily Saunders, of the hospice movement, uncovers a further attitude of considerable significance when she speaks of time for people being measured in quality rather than in quantity (du Boulay, 1984). How quickly can a doctor relate at depth? Must he spend time 'getting to know' the patient? Doctors need to be prepared to deal with the problems people bring and the feelings those problems represent, at the level the patient is at. That is the patient's need, and doctors both can, and must, go straight to the patient's level if they are to engage adequately with the problem the patient is working on. Those with a burning problem will not have come with the priority of getting to know the doctor for, as it were, a cup of tea and a social event. They have come, with some urgency, to understand themselves in a situation in which they feel caught and to get down to work. Talk in the consultation must necessarily be immediately at the level and depth at which the patient is struggling and quite regardless of how well the two know each other. The patient's work is on-going. They are well into it already. The doctor can therefore move in at depth even on a first consultation. The patient needs the doctor to move closer than would be the case in a social situation, and adjusts his boundaries to the doctor because of his temporary need and because it is a working relationship.

Lastly, the two following situations throw up interesting and important issues in relation to doctor's attitudes.

Nancy Friday (1981) describes a somewhat convoluted story that took place in North America. She tells of a newly-married couple having the wife's parents to lunch. The husband was carving a leg of lamb and was surprised to find that his wife had cut off the 'knuckle' of the leg before she cooked it. As he had not seen this done before he asked her why she had done it. She said she had always seen it done that way and referred to her mother. Mother, too, agreed she had always done the same and remembered, in her turn, that her mother had done so before her. Was there some special reason for this particular cooking habit in the bride's family? There was sufficient interest for them to bring this up when they next telephoned the bride's grandmother. Grandma, however, at first disagreed, saying she did not cut the knuckle off, but then, knowing that she very rarely had lamb, recalled that many years before, and when her daughter had been visiting one Thanksgiving Day, she had cooked lamb. It was an occasion when she was temporarily in a small flat with a small oven and she had cut off the thin, boney end of the leg in order to get the joint into the oven. This one occasion was what the bride's mother remembered and automatically repeated, and this behaviour had been unthinkingly reproduced through successive generations.

Here was a situation where habits had been formed through mistaken understandings, and only by questioning and putting things into words could behaviour be changed and the next generation freed to choose to cook the whole leg of lamb, or remove the knuckle, just as they wished. The doctor's work today can be seen to spread down through the generations increasing the offspring's flexible response to life. The effects of his work stretch out into the community, far outside the consulting room, and to people he may never meet. This experience may be worth remembering when movement in a patient's attitudes seems painfully slow, or the doctor's work is devalued and, as a consequence, he finds himself dispirited or inclined not to bother.

The second situation is the quite common one of the 'splitting' dynamic by a patient fascinatingly described by Tom Main (1968), and which relates to patients who split the medical team. This often occurs, for example, when a patient makes one doctor feel he is special to their care, while maintaining that another professional cannot do the job so well. 'But doctor, it's only you that seems to understand me', or 'Doctor, men don't really understand women's problems.' The team needs to compare notes and prevent this 'setting up' of one doctor against another from taking hold. The professionals must all work together if they are to challenge and protect themselves from this defensive behaviour. The real world that lies outside the internal fantasies of patients is not like that, and yet such is the strength of the patients' belief in their fantasies about people being all good or all bad, totally helpful or hopelessly useless, that it is important for the medical team to talk together and maintain themselves as a team of skilled people, each with their own relevant insights and abilities, and all of potential use to the patient in their different ways.

However, a doctor's ability to discuss his work openly and to involve himself in a team is a measure of his own development. Initially, shared discussion will often focus on some analysis of figures, and only later does it develop into sharing cases and, with time, move to the doctor's feelings about his work. When he does become able to discuss his work in a personal way, his own development progresses apace, and this in turn enables his patients to make healthy growth to further maturity (Mattinson, 1979).

I am aware, as I write, of the excess workload that most doctors have, and that all I write may therefore be met with scepticism and a belief that what I am describing can only increase their burden. There is often a belief that the more a doctor gets into problems with patients, the more work he does and the greater the time it will take. Yet, clearly, part of the doctor's role is to pick and choose an effective focus for his work, and he has the choice of whether or not to give time to any one patient. It is important to select patients appropriately. There are a whole variety of effective methods and different levels at which work with patients can be undertaken, and a doctor must feel free to choose how far he wishes to be involved and to judge the method and level that seem most appropriate to them both. It is valuable for him to be aware of the professionals in the community to whom he can refer patients he does not choose to work with – for whatever reason. In one-off consultations, patients will benefit from an accurately selected focus that attempts to penetrate to the heart of their problem. This takes perception and skill, but not necessarily any more time. In the numerically smaller number of carefully selected patients whom the doctor chooses to work with more fully, I am clear that ongoing, accurately focused work, taking more time and effort in the relatively short term of, say, three months will, in the longer term, both save him time and considerably increase his effectiveness and sense of achievement. In this context it must be remembered that a doctor will usually be in a practice for twenty-five years or more.

And the alternatives? A doctor can collude with a patient, stopping change and joining his patient in their boredom down the years. A patient may choose to see a doctor because he is not challenged, but rather, is colluded with in a defence system that protects him from the change and development he fears, but which also prevents a fuller, more effective life. Either the doctor and patient – their boundaries rigid and high – can hold each other at a distance so that their work together is largely ineffective; or – the boundaries of their feelings and personalities undefined – they can become enmeshed in each other's areas of responsibility, both confused and each locking the other in a merry-go-round, going nowhere.

CHAPTER 13

Doctors in Partnership

This chapter moves the focus of study from the relationships between patients and doctor to those between the doctors in a partnership. Partners usually meet on a daily basis and must plan and negotiate how they will undertake their work. Far too often there are competitive or controlling power plays that are undermining and stressful. When this is the case, those involved often seem to be stuck in their behaviour even though the grinding-down effect on the participants and their colleagues is there for all to see. The lives of the doctors, their families, the staff and even of the patients, will all be affected adversely and, at the same time, the doctor's efficiency is reduced by the resulting burn-up of emotional energy. Unnecessary stress and weariness are added to the lives of everyone concerned. While undoubtedly partner relationships can be a source of pleasure and good feeling, projections will play their part in doctors' lives as much as in any other groups. This subject is therefore arguably just as important as any other aspect of medical practice.

I must first admit that I have found relationships with partners quite difficult over the years and have only slowly become aware of the deep satisfactions and pleasures that lie amongst the difficulties. As support and fun have come more to the fore it has been as if the difficulties have stepped back into line and become less intrusive.

Relationships between partners are often thought to be difficult to study as many doctors consider them to be private. This assumption of the necessity of privacy makes it harder for a doctor to make comparisons with the norms of behaviour in the company boardroom. However, discussions down the years with doctors from a wide variety of practices have shown me that I have been far from alone in my difficulties, and confirmed that partner conflicts are a major source of stress. It is therefore pertinent to pose the question: 'What can the individual doctor do that will enable good working relationships?' This is a subject that clearly involves quite complex issues, but are there some vital seeds from which sound working relationships grow?

While in Canada I was told of the way the Iroquois Indians traditionally make their decisions. For their powwows they use a central ring from which a number of rawhide thongs radiate. Each thong is of equal length and there is one for each family representative. The powwow cannot begin until each thong is held: everyone must be present. They all sit in a circle, all equidistant from the centre – and each, of course, with a different perspective on the central ring – while they hear the concerns and ideas of each member. This symbolizes that everyone has a different view of the central issue, that all views hold equal validity and relevance and, unless those views are known and given due weight, a rounded and comprehensive decision cannot be made. That is the only type of decision they consider acceptable.

The attitudes encapsulated in this Iroquois Indian model are also pertinent to medical practices. Everyone is different; that is the happy and enriching reality, and that is how it should be. There is no place for the simplistic view that a decision will lie between what is either right or wrong, nor that everyone should have exactly the same aims, concerns and viewpoint. For instance, Belbin (1981), discussing teamwork, lists the characteristics required in a team of management and the different roles that individuals play: co-ordinator, plant (or ideas man), teamworker, shaper, specialist, implementer, evaluator, completer and resource investigator. Each of these skills is needed if a group is to work well and, of course, if an individual is gifted with one aptitude he almost certainly won't have some other, and while different people fulfil different roles, each must hold a different variety of concerns and priorities. Just because all the partners will be dissimilar and must inevitably hold divergent roles in the group, each needs the other's view point for the group to function well. The quality of the end point to their work depends on the group's ability to enable negotiation from all their different starting points – and conflicts are part of the package. They must be accepted and brought to the surface if everyone's concerns are to receive due weight. All members of the group hold a responsibility to ensure that each person is heard and that their concerns are included in the decision-making process. How this is handled is a responsibility that lies with the group rather than an individual or chairperson, and it determines how full and effective their working relationships will be.

A background necessity in working relationships must surely be an attitude in the members that they expect and allow adaptation to the ever-changing circumstances of the partners and the practice, along with an ability to learn, not only factually, but both by adjusting perceptions and attitudes, and by allowing experimentation with altered behaviour (Peters and Waterman, 1984). There is a model of the learning process that represents it as a spiral. People tend to focus on some area of interest until they have grasped it and applied it to a working end-point. They then move on to another concern. After a period of time they return to the first area of interest, but things have now developed and progressed; so the process can be best represented by a spiral rather than a circle. This is a simple and useful model: nothing is fixed; partners may agree some method to be tried, but it is always open for review. I sense that partnerships in ongoing difficulties – as opposed to the normal ups and downs of life – have not taken care of the learning spiral and of their personal developmental need for review and change. They become stressed and defensive and, as a result, less able to adapt.

There must be a multitude of reasons why people become defensive, but being over-stressed is a fairly universal cause and unfortunately it is all too common. People use many different defensive behaviours so as to maintain fixed systems, but most involve a withdrawal from real communication and, as a result, misunderstandings become common, have longer lives and result in frustration and anger.

Some people, when they are defensive, use change itself as a defence. In that case, the result of the change on the group is irrelevant: their personal gain gives the motive, and these motives (for instance, to display ability and gain kudos, or to grasp power) can be hidden. But this sort of behaviour has a manic, ungrounded feel and, while outwardly it is at the opposite extreme to the defence of undue fixity, it is similarly maladaptive and stressful. Effective change is open and honest in its intent and grounded in reality. It takes into account everyone's views and involves a solid negotiation that gives a sense of considerable satisfaction.

I wonder if the word 'negotiate' strikes you as it once did me. I remember a series of seminars on human development. There were presentations and discussions based on Erikson (1977) and Kegan (1982), on the baby, the infant and the teenager. Then the focus moved on to adulthood, and the presenter of that first seminar said, 'Well, adulthood is all to do with the ability to negotiate.' Just that. 'What? That's it? This is a cop-out. This member of the seminar has not bothered to prepare their presentation.' But over the succeeding weeks there followed some most fruitful and important discussions which seem, with time, to have touched on most aspects of adult interaction and yet indeed seem to be summarized simply by the word 'negotiation'.

There are so many ways to negotiate. For a child it is who has the biggest, or the fastest or the strongest that seems to be important and, no doubt, underlying this is the question of who is boss. Some adult organizations and managers also miss the real point and play power games: 'I'm paying you to do it my way.' But at its best, negotiation enables an energizing freedom for the participants. It takes account of each person's inner world, the way they see things and what is important to them – something that may have very little to do with fact and much to do with feeling. As such, negotiation is very much a mature person's ability and skill. A medical practice will make changes much more fruitfully if its members develop their negotiating skills. This will bear closer examination.

It would be useful to first consider an example. A frequent source of conflict in partnerships arises from workload comparisons. Rather than give time to discussing how they work and their attitudes to patients which demand a particular style, time is only given to a comparison of numbers. Some years ago a partner had taken on work outside his practice which involved him in a size-able and irregular time commitment. Sometimes this was in the evenings but usually for different periods in the day. Then one of his partners discovered that he fairly regularly spent time at his home during working hours. When casually asked where he had been, he would say that he had had to go off for this other work and had not therefore been able to take on a share of the home visits, etc. Attempts to clarify what was happening only resulted in defensive statements along the lines that all the partners had agreed to his taking on this extra work and had known it commit-ted him to irregular times out of the practice. He also emphasized that the financial reward for the extra work was shared by all the partners and the practice work he would otherwise have done must be taken off him. Suspicion and anger increased, but it seemed difficult to say so as there was an attitude, shared by all the partners, that it was not 'nice' to show suspicion, and they were all fearful of their anger, however gently verbalized. As a result silent, smouldering distrust became the underlying daily background to work.

The partner who discovered the other's behaviour became clear that continuing to avoid facing up to what was happening had become destructive of good relationships. This realization was in itself an important step for him and, he judged, made it impera-tive that he now do something. He decided to try and understand what was happening. To his surprise he began to perceive that the pressure of work, which he and his partners experienced, was not all patient- or work-generated, and was not therefore all a necessary and integral part of being a doctor. He recalled that he had been brought up by parents who were keen for him to 'succeed'. This, he now saw, had resulted in a pressured upbringing. He had taken on his parents' pressure for him to be always busy, to do it better, and to 'put more into it or he would not succeed'. He discovered that he only considered himself to be behaving adequately if he pushed himself to do more and more, and better and better. He did not set himself actual hurdles to clear, or achievable aims, but always considered he must 'do better'. 'Do better' had replaced 'be effective'. His normal and persistent state had become one of being on a treadmill. It was an exhausting, uncomfortable existence and now he also saw that it was quite unnecessary, because he enjoyed his work and in fact he was usually effective.

He began to see that not only did he pressurize himself with his attitudes but also pressurized his partners, because he expected that they, too, 'should do better'. But the effect he had on the partnership went even deeper, in that he had been involved in choosing some of his partners and had selected them because they also had the same 'good' perfectionist attitude to work. As a result, not only did he pressurize himself unnecessarily but also he had chosen a practice and partners who did so too. Then he also began to see that the pressures he experienced from his work were only in part realistic and that his own, separate, attitudinal pressures could never be satisfied. They were undefinable and unreal. They were also unpleasant and unnecessary. With this new perception he found his own attitudes were changing and, for instance, he began to allow respect and concern for his own feeling of being overworked. Through valuing his own feeling he discovered a concern for those of his partners', so that he no longer expected factual proof. Self-awareness, he decided, would play a far more important part in his life. From now on feelings would be given a firm place and carry due weight alongside the more factual workloads in the discussions at meetings with partners.

Beside this attitudinal change there were others. For a variety of reasons the increased number of home visits that had to be covered, with one partner away doing outside work, had tended to fall on him. Because of this, he had at first seen it as basically his problem that his partner was sometimes spending time at home, but he now reminded himself that all the partners had agreed to the outside work and they all took a share of the resulting remuneration. An equitable sharing of work was clearly the responsibility of all the partners, and so it was relevant to ask them what the partnership would do to equalize the extra work he felt had mostly fallen on him. Their workload management and shares were not a problem for him alone. They would all have useful views on the matter.

There are two things here of particular significance. First, by seeing it as a partnership problem rather than just his own, he drew in the less emotionally affected partners and immediately removed it from being a personal issue. The discussions were then less likely to arouse defensiveness and called on everyone's organizational responsibility rather than leaving it to him. Secondly, the focus he chose was on the factual effects of the extra work commitment rather than on his suspicion of the partner's dishonesty. He was choosing to discuss first something that was least personal as a way into the subject. He had given considerable thought to selecting which factors were most likely to be of mutual interest and cause least defensiveness, so as to be more likely to gain a flexible response.

Interestingly, what came out of the discussions (because in the event this did enable the problem to be well discussed) was that the doctor who had taken on the outside work had indeed begun taking time out in lieu of some of his extra evening commitments. He had done this without general consultation as he had not felt able to raise the issue with all the partners, but it transpired that he had in fact talked it over with one partner whom he considered particularly understanding and who had suggested he do exactly this, rather than admit to the rest of the partners that he was over-committed. These two had a common bond in being older than the rest, and each had begun to support the other in attempts quietly to preserve their waning energies, rather than openly admit the effects of their age. With this out in the open, honest negotiations could proceed. Clearly all parties had been less than open. He himself had not been prepared to acknowledge the degree of his annoyance for fear of his anger being considered 'out of control' and 'unprofessional'. The partner with the extra job had sought to keep his stress levels private because he saw them as resulting from being 'weak', and the sympathetic, older partner had secretly colluded in his taking time at home, adding a further deception. Each compounded the other's silence by adding their own. What was important in breaking through the deadlock was the one partner's increasing awareness of the importance of his feelings and the care taken to select a focus likely to be acceptable and, therefore, effective in opening up the discussion.

This may seem a trivial example and yet it was the source of very real emotions, and it serves to illustrate a lot of aspects that are common in partnership difficulties. Often members are held back from open communication and negotiation by a fear of offending others, or there can be a fear that to take the initiative in these situations (which are so often surrounded by the inertia of anxiety), is to risk being seen as disruptive, or even that there might be some resulting retribution. Not uncommonly there are secrets held by some members which are sealed by collusions and have been entered into for a variety of self-centred reasons. These members' shame then makes them defensively secretive and their collusion stubbornly obdurate, and yet secretiveness can only be confusing to those not in the know. They find it impossible to make sense of what is happening and must cope with the discomfort of being excluded from – they know not what. Not knowing, they build fantasies that are often bigger than the reality and which, in turn, are also kept private, further blocking understanding and proper communication. But whatever the characteristics of secrets, they are always destructive of the less stressful, more effective, more pleasant and collaborative ways of working. Any sub-group that holds information secret from the rest, or indulges in private decision-making or power play, should be clear that, in the longer term, their behaviour is destructive to the workings of the full group, and that that destructiveness is of a group or team that includes themselves.

What does effective communication in negotiation entail? For simplicity, consider two-person negotiation. What needs to happen, for instance, if you and I are to negotiate? Each of us needs to decide inside ourselves what it is we want: right down inside us and at gut level, what are our basic individual wishes from which all our detailed hopes develop? For some, this knowledge may come easily, but for others it is hard to find. Nevertheless, it needs finding. There may be pros and cons and considerable ambivalence, yet we need to weigh our thoughts and feelings and end up with our own clarity.

An example will help to show how important this can be. Right at the beginning of my sabbatical in Canada, I was looking for an apartment for the year. Imagine, then, a bewildered and rather lost man, unused to being away from his wife, family and friends, taken in by a friend of a friend and being trailed around by his wife with their two small sons. It was very humid and the temperature, day after day, was in the high eighties. We spent a week viewing a long succession of accommodations from the downright dreadful to the good but too pricey. But at last we found something that was not only good but also in the right price range, and with great relief we went down to the superintendent's office to sign the papers for the year. And I found I could not. What was going on in me? My companion was in despair. 'But John, this is almost exactly what you have been looking for.' I needed space to explore my confusion. We excused ourselves and went to a McDonald's for coffee.

Slowly I began to see that for me this was the point of no return. It was as if this year's sabbatical was suddenly no longer a fun spree, a sort of grand holiday: suddenly this was a whole year without my wife and sons. Once I had perceived where the feelings came from, I could weigh up this larger – and now focused – situation and become free to sign for the apartment. My head was saying, 'sign', but my feelings were making it impossible. Each needed to be considered and understood before I could function. Human thoughts and feelings are often described for convenience as if they are separate entities and yet we are indivisible and must function as an integrated whole. Attempts to avoid doing so risk maladaptive behaviour.

In negotiation, therefore, it is necessary to respect and understand oneself, one's past, present and hopes for the future, as well as to know and use all the three parts of the personality – the mind, emotions and abilities. We know ourselves if we are aware of all these: it is as if our spirit is alive, we can know what we want, can communicate the why and wherefore, and are well set to negotiate. And if we know and respect these aspects of ourselves, we will also be more aware and able to respect them in other people: each can hold his own power and no one attempts to set himself up as master. There is acceptance without manipulation. There can be an honest searching for a mutually satisfying solution through any differing needs.

To arrive at this point of awareness and understanding one, or both of us, may first need to discuss our thoughts and feelings in order to discover accurately what our wishes are. If we trust each other we can do this with one another; if not, we will need to go elsewhere to discuss it. The more we are able to trust, the more we are able to discover our wishes in an open way. Each can then understand where the other is coming from and both will be in a position to gain respect for the importance of specific issues for the other. No one makes himself into a doormat and neither uses the other as one. Each looks after his own wishes, but with regard for the other.

And yet it can be difficult to express our needs and wishes one to the other. For instance, if I am open with you and reveal my 'weakness', you might use that to bargain hard as a result. Deep in me I need to be able to trust; trust, on the one hand that you will speak your mind and, on the other, that you will respect my openness. We need trust that each will respect the other; trust that our individual, internal ways of understanding and considering things will be considered and valued.

Trust is not blind, nor does it involve one person doing what another expects of him. Lao Tsu, in the *Tao Ching*, records the four-thousand-year-old Chinese saying, 'He who does not trust will not be trusted' (Lao Tsu, translation 1973). Clearly, as this is Chinese wisdom, the opposite will also hold: that those who are able to trust will in turn be trustworthy.

It is indeed hard for one person to maintain his preferred self in the presence of extreme control or distrust. I suspect trust is to do with the individual's personal development, as trust of others must surely develop out of trust in oneself; from an acceptance, for instance, that this is the way I am, this is how I find myself, these feelings and thoughts are mine and, however confused or contradictory, I can live with them while I am still working on them. Meanwhile I am able to share them because of my own acceptance and, if I can trust myself in this way, it encourages others to do the same.

Once each of us has arrived at an understanding of what we feel about the issue, negotiation itself can begin, but the way in which we negotiate will often have its roots in our early experiences in our families of origin. Someone, for example, brought up in a large family where each child had to fight for what it got, may have little experience of any other option of behaviour than that of being highly competitive and pressurizing. Similarly, someone brought up as a single child in a family where Dad was never around and where the child therefore had Mum all to itself, may find it very hard to share. At its most extreme this experience can result in the child never experiencing a sharing of two people's viewpoints and as a result never developing an ability to look back: to reflect and 'play' with other people's ideas (Wilner, 1990) – clearly a severe handicap. Yet someone else, brought up to have his own way, may always expect his own agenda and preferred outcomes to be followed. People with little variety of experience in their upbringing other than these may need a considerably firm response, and to be given generous helpings of what it feels like to have to live with their behaviour if they are to become more self-aware and considerate people. And in some families there will have been much demanding jealousy, greed or envy. The ways in which individuals behave with others is profoundly affected by their early life experiences in the first small group of their family of origin. Recurrent, painful behaviour experienced in the past will unconsciously be assumed likely to recur, and defenses appropriate to the past can be reactivated automatically, although in their new situation these may be totally inappropriate. For instance, a partnership of doctors, who may be very nice people as individuals, can, as a result of their membership of the partnership group, perform quite destructively while being amazingly unaware of the effect they are having. Happily, behaviour can be observed and the group's dynamics used to move it over to being helpful. Basically one's own interventions need choosing in the light of their likely effect. In situations like this a course in the formal study of groups can hold rich rewards.

So negotiation takes place between the two of us, and of course there are many possible end-points. One happy situation is when we both find we want the same end-point. Expression of one's own wishes is then happily matched by the other's, and the negotiation culminates with satisfaction on both sides. But this satisfaction can only happen if there has been a process of open discussion. Often it is assumed that open discussion has taken place when actually it has not.

Frequently, though, there will not be an immediate match of wishes, and then there are a whole range of end-points that lie on a continuum that extends from you having things entirely as you wish (and me having what I least wish), all the way through to the reverse positions. Full discussion, which includes the feeling level, makes agreement here much easier, because if the background feelings and thoughts have been shared, each is helped to make compromises or to decide whose preference matters most this time. The warmth of closeness can be a recompense for my agreeing to your preference this time, and the ongoing nature of the relationship means that each may have a turn at being less than fully pleased.

So much for negotiation between two people. But this atmosphere of creative negotiation is of even more importance in the larger forum of a partnership where the concerns and differing views of several partners must be taken into account, and where the conflicts within each individual are in addition to those between the partners and multiplied by the size of the partnership. It is clearly right and inevitable for conflicts to abound. They are best placed openly on the table for everyone to understand, respect and consider before attempts are made to reach any decisions. Instead they are often feared and conflict denied, or the issues brushed aside as if conflict holds danger. It is, however, a necessary stage in a process towards a balanced end-point. 'Getting on' with other people includes confrontation and facing difference, rather than sidestepping it, or insisting on everyone apparently being the same.

It will be worthwhile considering all this by approaching it from a different viewpoint. At first it may seem to the reader that the subject has been changed but it will later become clear that it has not. What I wish to show is the value of the group's members taking the individual's personalities into account as they negotiate. For this it will help to consider the characteristic of assertiveness, and the extremes of aggression and submission. An assertive stance is usually seen as lying on a continuum between the other two extremes.

Submissive people tend to withdraw when there is disagreement; they become uninvolved and keep their views to themselves. To this end they may pretend agreement rather than put forward their concerns (which might be to risk disagreement). It can be surmised that they unconsciously believe that in this way their past experiences, perhaps of repetitive, bruising onslaughts from an aggressive and intrusive parent, have resulted in a wish never to impose such an experience on others. It may be that they even fear being tainted with any characteristic that might remotely be seen as having an aggressive effect on those around them and, as a result, are reluctant to put forward their point of view in case it might put pressure on someone else; but in doing this, it is as if they themselves become hidden and lost. Indeed, they may not even know their own point of view as, not knowing it, there is no possibility of it being perceived and, therefore, of their being seen as even remotely challenging. It is as if their concern not to be manipulative or overbearing makes them too anxious to be able to function as the persons they are. They will agree to anything so as not to have to bear either the anxiety that difference with others produces or the possibility of their needs pressurizing someone else. Effectively, however, they are immobilized by their anxiety. (This is of course describing an extreme, but others may have these anxieties to a lesser, and yet debilitating, degree.)

There are responses other than that of submission which a child might make to an overbearing and intrusive parent. For instance, he might unconsciously choose to respond with aggression. If people are seen as a threat, their advances would then result in defensive parries and thrusts to prevent any closeness. At some level everyone longs for sharing and closeness, but in these children repetitive experience has taught them that that would be likely to involve a further episode of being trampled upon. Safer, then, to keep other people at a distance.

It is possible to surmise, therefore, that a child whose trust has been shaken by persistent aggression will be defensive, and the most obvious defences are those of submissively hiding away or of aggressively keeping others at a distance. In either case the defensive behaviour may become continuous, even though, with time and changed circumstances, that may no longer be appropriate or necessary. In effect the child loses his ability to move out from his defensiveness to the median behaviour of being 'normally' assertive.

But, interestingly, the same two end-points may result from the opposite childhood experience: that of an upbringing with an overly retiring parent who is unavailable to the child. These children may develop the same fearful inability to allow closeness which their parents displayed. It is as if such a child mirrors the parent's unexplored fears, picking them up and taking them on himself while unaware of their cause. Or, conversely, the child may learn to chase after the emotionally unavailable parent and become aggressively intrusive in a vain attempt to make contact. It is as if such a child overstates and presents himself so as to be sure to make plain that he is clearly available. He may even remorselessly pursue other people, as if he has learnt to expect that all relationships roll away into crevices between the bare floorboards of his life.

Therefore we can speculate further that, whether a child has invariably experienced the extreme of aggression or of submission, he may respond with either of those same extreme behaviours himself.

These last paragraphs have been an attempt to gain some insight into the possible childhood developments of these defensive behaviours. What, though, of these children when later, as adults, they come up against aggressive personalities? As adults they may again find themselves pulled and pushed into extreme behaviours. Aggression makes some people also fly to aggression as a defence, while others become numbed and shocked, defensively retreating into a passive submission.

Unfortunately, both these extreme responses only serve to confirm an aggressor in his behaviour but, of course, we are now considering the responses of adults who can think and plan to function in different ways. Adults have the option of varying their defence if they consciously think the situation through. What is needed, when first faced by aggression, is for all concerned to remain themselves; to gently but firmly maintain their own person and not allow themselves to be squashed into submission or forced into aggressive, verbal fighting. The adult, far more than the child, can choose to vary his defensive stance to one designed to draw a more appropriate and useful behaviour out of the other person. The skill is to remain oneself; to work to remain one's own outgoing, open, warm self, and so disarm the aggressor while at the same time being secure in the faith that at some level everyone's desired norm is of course to be outgoing and warm.

To do otherwise is to hold and maintain the other person in

144

their ineffectual, fixed, aggressive mode and to make it difficult for him to move away from it into a flexible, ever-adjusting and, therefore, ever-relevant way of being.

The main point to this foray into developmental and systems theories is that each partner bears a share of responsibility for the system of behaviour into which they are all locked, and it is therefore everyone's responsibility to change his own part in the unfortunate and ineffective way of interacting with each other. To make one person a scapegoat, by blaming him for the way the group functions, is only to draw attention away from one's own equally unhelpful, undesirable and dysfunctional part in the collusion that has made the group what it is. If a partner is aggressive, the rest of the doctors in the practice can hold him in his aggressive behaviour, they can maintain him in that stance and make it difficult for him to slip easily into another way of being. They themselves may have slipped into their old-style playground or tribal defence of isolating someone who is different, rather than the adult way of speaking out to make him uncomfortable in his unfortunate behaviour, pointing out the need to change to something more likely to be effective. A change in attitude in those around an aggressive partner is needed if a recurrent, undesirable situation is to change.

If each member is responsible for his own behaviour and also for his share in the way the system functions, then it only takes one person consistently to alter his own stance for the balance of the group to shift and for a new equilibrium to develop or, preferably, to move the group to a flexible system. Each member is able to alter the system by himself taking responsibility for his part in whatever it is in the practice that offends him.

Here an example will help, both to lend clarity and to draw together the various strands. I will take the fairly common situation in family practice: that of the hallowed 'senior partner syndrome'. It has been remarkable to me how often this situation has been the source of pervasive distress that has been brought to case discussion groups down the years. Not only does the discomfort of these situations affect the partners, but it pervades all they do, so that it even inhibits their work with their patients: it is so invidious!

The senior partner in these practices is a man who maintains a rigid defence against his anxieties. He holds to his own ideas and aggressively parries other people's (and sometimes an apparently passive stance is actually very aggressive). Control seems to be all important to him, otherwise his fears would know no bounds. While his defence was perhaps appropriate to some past situation, it has outlived its usefulness, and as long as his control is unchallenged by the partners, he does not discover the current ground-less nature of his fear. Meanwhile he quietly poses on a pedestal labelled 'Power' or 'Control', projecting his impotence onto those around him. It is sad to see him: it stultifies the partnership and everyone is frustrated.

Meanwhile, his colleagues may seem free to speak their minds. 'He likes to be in control.' 'We all know what is needed, but the senior partner won't let us do that.' He is blamed for many of the problems in the system, yet it is a system in which each partner plays their part.

It can be difficult for the partners to enter into this. They probably sense the older man's vulnerability, but in reality that only means that his fears will need sensitive consideration, not a frozen inactivity. It may be that the partners pick up his fear but perceive it as their own fear of his rounding on them, and shrink from a possible re-enactment of some past degrading experience at his hands. But if constraints such as these do operate, the other partners can remind themselves that they are adults, that the issues involved are dear to their own hearts, and that any short-term discomfort will bring considerable long-term gain to all members of the partnership which will ultimately be to the ben-efit of staff and patients too. Before becoming a partner, young doctors may well have felt that a written reference and future jobs depended on their behaviour towards more senior colleagues, but this no longer applies once they are secure in a partnership. In-deed, if a young doctor will enter into the more difficult areas of partner relationships, he makes himself indispensable.

What other attitudes make it so difficult? Often there is a problem that lies in the age differences. Younger partners, per-ceiving the older man as a parental figure, hold an attitude that the older man has an authority to be controlling. Certainly a child has no right to equality nor is it able to challenge its parents on equal terms, and the child does indeed depend on the parent for support, encouragement and financial aid. Until such time as an adult perceives himself as having ability and adult status alongside an older man and, as a result, can shake off the transference of his childhood feelings for his parents from the older partner, it can be hard to hold an expectation of equality. An adult stance would be one where the individual respected himself as the adult he is while at the same time perceiving the senior partner as merely holding a role; a role which is to function openly for the good of the partners and the practice.

But what can the partners do in this type of situation?

No one can disagree with statements that come from the heart and speak of an individual's feelings. 'I am feeling frustrated with the way we seem unable to make reasonable change in the practice. We are five adult, concerned, able doctors, and the individual problems of each one of us warrant consideration. For my part, I don't feel that we offer this to each other.' 'It often seems that we treat each other very competitively, and that the energy we expend on that would be better turned outwards onto our competitors, leaving us free to collaborate. Collaboration between us would be more efficient, more creative and satisfying, and certainly less stressful.' 'I am finding I am too stressed for too much of the time and, from what I see of the rest of you, we all are. It makes me feel dispirited. I am sure we can find other, more pleasant ways to work. It is surely true that if doctors are happier and less stressed, then their patients will also have a better service.' 'The things I find most difficult are ... and I need to discuss them. It would help me to know how you all handle this', etc.

There would need to be something more consistent than, for instance, one single outburst followed by retreat into ineffectual submission. There would be the discomfort that comes with any unsettling of a rigid system; a short-term rocking of the boat for the sake of the longer-term good (and a partnership does go on for many years). 'Rocking the boat' is often portrayed as a 'bad' thing, but a boat cannot be sailed purposely forward unless it is held to the wind, and it heels and rocks just because it is straining forward.

For there to be a change in a partnership requires a change of attitude in only one partner initially. That is the starting point. It requires an attitude that maintains a stance of the expectation of a reasonable adaptation to the needs of everyone affected. The attitude will include concern and respect for each member: junior partner, receptionist, office clerk, cleaner, the patients and, of course, oneself. It will include respect for the senior partner so that he is included in discussions rather than talked about behind his back and labelled as, for instance, 'controlling', yet not told about the effects of this on the partners and on the work of the partnership. Isolation and sniping can only result in his keeping up the drawbridge that divides 'them' from 'us' and keeps the partnership split into two defensive camps.

Respect for each person may also demand a different attitude to the partner who is quiet and retiring. His concerns and thoughts have an equal value and are required by the team if they are to have a full, rounded discussion and come to an effective end-point. A partner like this presents a challenge to the others:

the challenge of drawing out everyone's concerns before attempting to integrate them into agreements. The learning spiral is one of constant movement and no permanent fixity. It demands open discussion of all viewpoints before agreeing what to try next. It will be necessary for behaviour which blocks this full involvement of all the members to be acknowledged verbally; for instance, both aggressive or submissive behaviours would require open discussion by the group if ever they got in the way of effective group work.

Sometimes a partner may play the game of assuming knowledge of what another feels or wants, and will make decisions based on these assumptions. These people frequently consider themselves to be especially empathetic and considerate, but their assumptions only serve to control the situation, and arise out of an unbelievable arrogance. Each individual must be expected and allowed to consider, decide and speak for himself.

It is as if a primary challenge for the partners is to keep all their members within the team rather than to allow one member to split off by behaving aggressively or submissively, or indeed through any other consistent defensive behaviour. The team needs all its members to participate. They must work with care to include all their members. Each has different and valuable insights and abilities. There will inevitably be conflicts in the group's processes which will need containing rather than brushing aside. If one member needs help to be confrontational, so be it. If another needs help with his arrogance, so be it. If one needs help to be in touch with his feelings of impotence or sadness, so be it. Acknowledgement of feeling enables the individual to develop into a more balanced person and become a more versatile team member. It will help the team to discover and use the abilities of all its members and work more effectively. Most certainly there is a serious loss to the whole partnership whenever one partner's concerns are not met.

Finally, there is another important skill and service the doctor can develop for his partners. It can be seen as mirroring what he may do for patients. For example, a colleague tells me he finds that when he has had a bad night on call, perhaps with several disturbances or when he has dealt with a patient in a particularly distressing situation, he finds that partners (incidentally, both medical and marital) all tend to take the attitude: 'Well that's life: you are paid for it' or, 'Don't make a fuss: we too have the same sort of nights on call.' While these reactions hold truth – and he knows it – he is actually trying to discuss his feelings in relation to his work. He finds that no one acknowledges that it has been difficult for him; that he must be weary; that his patient's death must have been distressing for him. He does not want those feelings brushed aside as if they were nothing. He would value someone being there for him, just as he has been there for his patients.

It is as if this doctor's partners are all striving to prevent the distress of medical work insinuating itself further into their lives, as if they personally experience it as overwhelming, and fear and resent it. In an attempt to hold back the flood, they react by ignoring it in their colleagues, as if denying it will somehow make the other's stress go away. It is a vain attempt to stop work's tentacles spreading from doctor to doctor, or into the doctor's home, but unfortunately such behaviour only serves to distance them from the person who is stressed, making his situation worse. An ability to keep close to him by acknowledging his burden, will also allow discussion to seek ways that will help contain its invidious effect. And of course, what one person does for another today will in time be rewarded by the same skills being offered in return.

The essence of this is that partners be at ease with feelings. If they are not, they may create problems for one member by projecting their depressed feelings or their stress onto a sensitive colleague. On the other hand, if they are at ease with feelings, they can be of considerable service in freeing a doctor ensnared in the labyrinths of a patient's projected feelings. A partner who is aware of himself, and who is distanced from the situation with a particular patient, can enable that doctor to find a way out from projection's grip and back to his own reality. Time given by the partners to sorting feelings is well spent: it frees the doctor concerned, improves and speeds the work of the practice, develops mutual understanding and reduces everyone's stress levels.

Without feelings being considered and received by his colleagues, the doctor finds himself shutting off in his turn from the feelings of family and patients alike. Often he will then be horrified at himself, believing – and concerned – that he is losing his humanity. A doctor stays with his patients at considerable cost to himself and he in turn needs both to care for himself and to receive care from others. There is need for the complete circle. In a partnership, doctors can join in developing that full circle. The result can only be for the good of everyone concerned.

CHAPTER 14

The Search for Freedom

There is a theme running through this book like a thread: that people need to be free to be themselves and, in particular, that doctors must work to be as free as possible from patient projections and from projecting themselves onto patients. This chapter draws on psychotherapeutic understandings of human development and personality, to outline an underlying philosophy for the doctor's work that encompasses this belief and, at the same time, consolidates the description of the family doctor's psychological role. It brings the book round full circle, and of course the circle is itself an image which speaks of wholeness and inherent freedom of movement, free from the vertical and linear structure of unnecessary hierarchy and control.

An unexpected bonus in writing this book has been the opportunity to involve friends and colleagues in reading and discussing the manuscript and so discovering the variety of their reactions. This has been particularly intriguing with regard to the response to this particularly chapter. In general, people find it interesting, but some have enthused about it, saying it is the heart of the book and that it is of particular importance to them. Why should there be such a difference in reactions? Of course, people are not all the same, but it seems to me that for some people this chapter speaks to an inner conflict in a way that makes them feel deeply understood. Perhaps the difference is that some have a greater inner sense of security, are more free to be themselves and feel intrinsically more at home, while others must search for these qualities, find they must strive hard for space and air to breathe freely, and are highly sensitive to any gradient in their freedom or restriction in their environment.

It must surely be significant that today's young doctors seem to qualify and leave their medical schools dispirited by what they have come to know about the conditions in which medicine is now practised. The reduced numbers who elect to continue into their hospital jobs and so become fully registered doctors are often, quite frankly, depressed by their work, by the relentless hours, by their sense of working in isolation (or with colleagues who seem never to stop running), by an increasing number of patients who seem to view their relationship with their doctor as something that the doctor offers and in which they themselves play only a passive part, by a growing view that administrators and politicians seem to stand over and against them, rather than alongside, and by increasing restrictions on their freedom to speak out about any concerns they may have for the service they are striving to provide. Without doubt bureaucratic restrictions are growing year by year with little to show in the way of improved doctor/patient relationships (the heart of medicine), but rather in dissatisfaction and increasing pressure. As was said in a letter to *The Times* (18 August 1994), most patients do not, in fact, want the decision as to the best treatment for them to be made by a government minister, or by a health service manager or even by the doctor alone. They want to be part of a team of people who communicate well, who are up-to-date with the relevant medical issues, and who recognize that the people at the centre of the process of making decisions about their lives, are themselves (Watson, 1994).

In the same paper another letter points out the lack of real democratic legitimacy in the changes that have recently been forced upon the National Health Service, and states that major changes in our public institutions properly require public mandate, public consultation and public consent, whereas what was done to the National Health Service in the recent changes had none of these. In contrast the writer feels that what is now needed is the reviving of public confidence in the primacy of social purpose for the National Health Service and the restoration of a sense of ownership and responsibility for it; both in those who use it and those who work in it (Keen, 1994). Certainly for doctors the list of growing restrictions is long and their effects are broad and deep. There are restrictions on prescribing, on referral options, even on who will be treated, on how the doctor must arrange his work each week, on the selection of the courses he must attend each year, on performance measurements (by criteria that are not agreed) and on priorities for patient care that seem trivial, both to those who work directly with patients and to the patients themselves. There is now pressure that, in future, rates of pay should be determined by these extraneous performance measures, and this is made more sinister in that freedom of speech about the National Health Service is being restricted in new contracts of employment. At the same time doctors understand that administrators themselves are paid more if they make economies that pressure others to work harder and harder, and to work in ways that increase the figures of patients treated to the detriment of reasonable safety. They are told that doctors have had too much power in the past (and told so by those now seen to grasp it for themselves for its own sake). They are told that doctors must be accountable, meaning they must do as someone else dictates. However, that someone does not hold himself equally accountable to those other members of the team who work as frontline providers – the doctors and nurses. This results in the medical profession finding itself not only accountable to patients (which is important and onerous enough in itself), but also progressively to administrators, while no one is accountable to them in turn. They are held trapped ever more firmly as pigs-in-the-middle, with no sense of any reciprocal concern. In the past, the doctor's private time and personal life were frequently hostage to his work but now, progressively, so are his personal motivations and work practices.

If there are those who shrug their shoulders and say, 'Well, that's life in the 1990s', they should be reminded that over the centuries people have repeatedly come to believe that individuals are involved in a deep-rooted search for the freedom to be their own person. This search has been variously described in more recent times as: 'for autonomy'; 'for wholeness'; 'for individuation' (Jung, 1964), or 'to be that self which one truly is' (Kierkegaard, 1941). It is also as if society in general has a collective mind or unconscious (Jung, 1964), and struggles to see what it wants to be and where it wants to go, as if it has a shared philosophy of its own. And if all this is so, it must have special relevance to a doctor's work. It would mean the doctor's being conscious of this need in all individuals as he works, and so take care to encourage and nurture freedom for his patients. It would also mean that, if the doctor's own freedom 'to be' were to be taken hostage, the process would be acutely stressful. Meanwhile, however, in reality, human values today seem to be losing to the principles of monetarism, and to what can be bought.

But is freedom so important? Brian Keenan, as the world knows, was kidnapped by the Islamic Jihad in Beirut and held hostage for four-and-a-half years. He has written of his ordeal (1992) and tells of how one day he heard the dreadful cries of a man being tortured, and when he was next taken to exercise in a larger room, found a pair of pliers beside bloodstains on the floor. He describes his dawning realization of the pliers' use and that if they had been used to abuse someone else, then it could well be his turn next. He believed he had a better purpose for the pliers and, by taking them, he would prevent their misuse. He writes of a need to hold onto freedom, however limited that freedom might be, and so he hid the pliers in his pants, willing to face the 'agonizing worry' that he might be discovered. This small act of personal choice and freedom brought him what was, he makes clear, an immensely important feeling of exhilaration. A small, defiant action brought him an inner escape from other people's control.

It is interesting how extreme situations serve to clarify the fundamentals, stripping the inessentials away. People who have described similar experiences of having been controlled and defiled also write of their need to hold onto this inner sense of freedom. It is as if one fundamental human requirement is for an independence that allows the human spirit's lungs to expand to their full capacity and, when outer freedoms are curtailed, they seem prepared to use their last breath in an awesome determination to hold onto this inner freedom.

One major thing that struck me out of many in Brian Keenan's book was the extraordinary analysis he makes of the inner freedom he and John McCarthy found, and the theory of projection which could in every detail have been taken from some textbook on the subject. I am sure it is no accident that this is so strikingly found in a book on the experience of being held hostage, a situation where there is a desperate need to hold onto sanity by casting off the jailor's projections and wrestling for freedom for oneself. And again and again in literature, as people tussle with what freedom is and how to attain it, pure projection theory seems to leap up out of the pages.

For instance, it is also very clearly found in John Fowles' novel, *The French Lieutenant's Woman* (1969), a novel portraying the experiences of a young man striving for the freedom to be himself as he moves into adult interrelatedness and the 'affectional bond of marriage' (Bowlby, 1979). His constraints are made more obvious by setting the novel in the mid-nineteenth century, with the extremes of formality and wealth so rife at that time. The same processes are clearly portrayed by Edith Wharton in *The Age of Innocence* (1974), a novel set in New York at about the same time, and when rigid, unwritten protocols reigned supreme in a society that attempted to protect and elevate itself but, in so doing, stifled and imprisoned the individual, impelling him more quickly to find an inner freedom.

Everyone, in every age and place, and whatever their social setting or form of work, must make this same personal journey for themselves, but the need is at its most acute whenever rules and society's expectations are at their most rigorous. Not only are the current health service changes stifling, but medical practice has long been heavily laced with the protocols, taboos and guidelines that have developed down the centuries and which have evolved to safeguard the patient's independence. Yet, while these may be referred to in medical schools, they are seldom discussed in a way that enables a doctor to make them his own. At the same time, those who turn to their doctors at times when they are ill and when their lives depend on medical skills, often have fixed, defensively-held expectations and requirements. These outer restrictions on their doctor's behaviour are at once mirrored and compounded by the more subtle, more personally powerful, internal processes of projection and projective identification, which require far more than an undiscussed rule of ethics to enable a doctor to function with an integration of thought and feeling. It is within this kind of atmosphere of restrictive, unspoken expectations and rigidly held assumptions, quite apart from the experience of being physically taken prisoner, that projections live most firmly and securely. Doctors especially can feel hostage to their work.

But even though viciously severe hostage ordeals are thankfully not those of the majority, everyone has the background experience of presumptuous and unspoken limitations on their freedom, so that at some level this experience will have been powerfully theirs. For instance, we have all been small, impotent children, slowly growing up and steadily demanding a release from adult controls that have not always kept pace with our fast-developing abilities and our desire to be free to try our wings. Parents do not always discuss these matters with their children as, no doubt, they judge the child too young to understand. A parent's attitudes, therefore, remain unspoken and often unintelligible to the child, while they can be experienced as being heavily restrictive.

It will be useful briefly to consider this childhood development process further. Erik Erikson (1977) analyses the stages of human development, and affirms that the phase at which the child begins to be responsible for himself coincides with his ability to control defecation. Responsibility for self may therefore first be worked out in relation to toileting. That being so, it is not surprising if bowel function and issues of control become linked in the human psyche.

Recently, a man told me of his wife's handling of a situation with their small daughter. The child had clearly needed to empty her bowels. Mother said, 'Do you want your potty, Sally?' Sally shook her head. 'All right', said mother, 'Tell me if you want me'. Sally went off into another room and a short time later appeared having messed her knickers. Uncritically, mother said: 'Let's go and clean you up, Sally.' That task done, mother and daughter had a loving cuddle before each got on with what interested them.

Father, telling me all this, was deeply moved by what he had witnessed. Here was a mother whose guiding principle was that she loved her daughter and this priority extended to allowing her freedom to be herself, to make her own decisions, and to have time to discover how she wished to organize herself. Mother had confidence in the process of learning, in the child's good sense, and in her right to find out and decide for herself. She held a guiding principle, or concept, that Sally was to be free to make her own choices and come to her own conclusions. As an individual, Sally was respected and left paramount in her own life, while mother's perception of how she hoped Sally would behave was not allowed to restrict the spirit of the developing child. Meanwhile, mother would see that nothing of any real importance would come to any harm and, no doubt, after a week or two, Sally did decide she would use the potty.

Of course, Sally's mother could have done differently. She could have decided unilaterally that it was now time Sally used her potty, and then, presumably, Sally would have been induced to sit on it whether or not she had reached the stage when she both could and wanted to cope. 'Come on, Sally, time you used your potty.' Mother's wishes, and Sally's wish of the moment, might well have been at variance and, if Sally did not perform to order, there would have been a feeling of mother's dissatisfaction hanging in the air between them. If, on the other hand, Sally had happened to be ready to perform, then there would have been a sense of her being good – but only because she had pleased her mother, rather than by her own ability to get her act together. How sad, by comparison, to the eventual feeling this mother enabled, of the child being in charge of herself.

The father recounting this family scene was distressed at the memories of his own upbringing which had had no similar guiding principle of the importance of autonomy. He considered that, in this regard, people entering adulthood (a time when they are rightly beginning to seek to fulfil their own needs) have different starting points as a result of their upbringings. And, of course, the attitudes surrounding a child in relation to potty training will be largely the same through all the other childhood journeys of self-discovery.

At the same time as the child is reaching for these external freedoms for itself, it is also gaining internal abilities. It is in the early days of infancy that a baby is enmeshed with its mother, using her to carry and sort out its projected feelings to such an extent that the mother may seem only an extension of the child (Winnicott, 1962). That stage does not last long and as the baby's increasing experience and maturity enable it to understand itself, so there is an increasing trust and use of its own feelings without first needing another person's participation. This must surely be the start of a person's real freedom which begins when children firmly own their inner feeling world and hold an inner independence.

No doubt the takeover from parental involvement in these processes will not be strictly in time with a child's developing abilities
and its need for the freedom to be itself and, as a result, children
come to see other people as responsible for curtailing their freedom.
Later on, despite changed circumstances and abilities, the young
adult may continue in this belief – and, of course, the unfortunate
reality is that some people do treat others in a highly controlling
manner that may serve to maintain the confusion.

In general terms this shift from infant dependency to independence will in many ways have become a conscious process by the
time of adolescence. If, for the moment, it is assumed that there
is nothing else happening in the young person's life, then the
adolescent's options might be seen to be between being childishly
dependent or being totally independent. There would be an all-
or-nothing conflict between, on the one hand, being involved with
others but sacrificing autonomy and, on the other, of being quite
separate from other people and so being completely independent.
And yet, although adolescent youngsters often have black-or-white
attitudes, this situation does not really exist in the world, and
much of what people do can only take place if they are involved
with others. For instance, I cannot have an interchange of ideas
that enables me to refine my own thinking unless I am open to
explore what someone else thinks. Nor can I focus on my own
area of interest unless others dig, sow and reap, so giving me the
time. I cannot experience being a father unless another will be a
mother and there is a child. Human development depends on the
individual being firmly rooted in society; his freedom 'to be' is
won, not by demanding a simplistic independence but rather by
diving headlong and deep into the waters of intimacy and interdependence.

Karen Horney has explored the conflict between independence
and interdependence (1946). The shift with increasing maturity to
interdependence, she states, requires inner changes and these she
summarizes as the abilities: 'to move towards people', 'to move
against them' and 'to move away from them'.

I want to fill out Karen Horney's three concepts and relate
them to one another.

As a teenager I used to go pot-holing (or caving) in the Men-
dip Hills in Somerset. I remember the first occasion at Swildens
Hole. It was not simply that my friend and I arrived at the cave
one day and went in. Far from it. We talked about the trip a
great deal: which pot-hole would we try? We read about them; we
discussed how many hours we could spend underground; we
weighed up the choice between a dry cave or one with water

running through, and we considered whether we wanted to scale a vertical section within the cave.

We made our final choice because we liked the idea of squeezing down into a pot-hole beside a surface stream that disappeared into the same small hole. It added a whole extra dimension in that it meant we needed to take the weather into account: if it rained while we were underground it would raise the level of the stream, making our exit impossible until such time as its swollen waters subsided. We also liked the idea that quite a long way into our chosen pot-hole there was a vertical section over which the stream cascaded and which would require a twenty-foot wire ladder and safety rope. Our pot-hole held multiple challenges, each bringing its own interest but each requiring preparation. My friend was reassured that I could tie a bowline knot to secure the top of the rope ladder and the safety rope around our waists. He, however, never quite got the hang of tying one himself.

And so our preparations went ahead. We arranged to borrow the necessary equipment, but there was also the preparation within ourselves for what we would face.

When the day came, we hitchhiked to the nearby village and changed our clothes in a barn. The stream, we discovered, ended in a pleasant pool overhung by trees, and the pot-hole itself formed the outflow from the pond. We were well pleased with the pleasant atmosphere of the place. It was a cold day with snow on the ground and we were getting cold. There is always an even temperature inside caves, so that in winter weather it is often warmer and more pleasant inside than out; so we quickly let ourselves slide, feet first, into the narrow, rocky cleft. I found the first thirty-feet or so quite unpleasant, because the noise of the rushing, tumbling water drowned any talk between us as we squeezed and groped our way through a narrow, water-splashed section with our eyes not yet adjusted to our torchlight. However, my friend said later that he had found that the resulting isolation gave him a sense of doing it alone, which pleased him.

Entry into a relationship can be looked on as if it were a pot-holing experience, a journey into the unknown or, as Karen Horney puts it, 'to move (in) towards people' and to become involved with others. People enter into relationships if they consider there is more to gain in than out, if they like the other person and if they believe they have an ability to endure the hazards they will face in the unknown dark: to resist cloying damp and cold, scale the difficult vertical climbs and survive intact, regardless of what they might meet. They need a belief in their ability to have times alone despite being with another, and yet to join in carrying ladders and ropes and the sharing of an ability to tie knots and other responsibilities. They need a belief that the experience will add something to them as people, and that at the end each will not merely have survived, but also feel invigorated. Finally, of course, they need to feel strong enough to move out of the situation if and when they wish, and to be able to cope with the feelings of loss and emptiness that inevitably result.

While some people develop from the isolation end of a whole spectrum of starting points, being unsettled and wary of even briefly receiving another's projections, others will move out from a state of fusion where projections abound to such an extent that it is as if the two have no boundaries and that each is inside the skin of the other and has no identity of his own. So it is that in some people the need to find an internal personal freedom is externalized in a search for isolation: for example, on mountain sides or sailing the oceans on their own – situations where they are well separated from people's enmeshing projections. Their internal needs seem to demand space, free from the perceived threat of intrusion. But for others, their externally reflected need is for an over involvement with others, even to so cling to another that there is no space between, as if they live off the other's feelings rather than find, and own, their own. Frequently there will be a mix of both extremes in the same person, though one will usually predominate (Symington, 1986). But whatever the state from which people start, there is a need in everyone to be able to draw close to others and yet at the same time to remain different. Without this ability, men and women are diminished, they lose out and deny themselves the opportunity for development. It demands all the skills that Karen Horney calls the 'ability to move against people'. It is the ability to rub up against others and not only survive but maintain one's own boundaries and be more finely honed in the process. It involves taking responsibility for oneself and for one half of the relationship, holding one's own feelings and negotiating, so as not to lose individuality but rather to enhance it; not to have to passively accept another's projections but to hear and understand about the other person's inner world of feeling – knowing it and experiencing it as quite separate to one's own. It is as if the boundaries of the self are defined, and with that definition comes both responsibility for oneself and freedom to be an individual.

It would seem from all this that, starting in infancy, people begin to own their inner world of feeling and, as a result, steadily develop their own understandings and sense of self. It is largely from this that the child becomes a separate, autonomous being. This process develops initially within the child's own family and within the small circle of that family's friends and acquaintances but, about the time of adolescence – a time when he chooses for himself who he will be with and where he will go and what he will do – he must continue this process in the outer, different world that is now defined by the adolescent's own choosing. Adolescent independence is often seen as the time of making a choice to leave the world which was chosen and defined by parents (and where reactions to it have often already been set down and are followed by force of habit and the offspring manipulated by parental expectation), and enter a new world whose boundaries are chosen by the adolescent, and where he can make his own individual and quite separate responses. In essence, the journey is one of developing interdependence with a group of the adolescent's own choosing, and in a way and at a level that he alone wishes. It demands an ability to have and sustain intimacy with others while maintaining his own person and individuality.

This maintenance of self must mean that, whatever the expectations and projected pressures within society, it is ultimately man's own inner beliefs and perceptions that lend a sense of wholeness. His freedom results from acceptance of himself with all his variety of feelings. This results in a state of increased awareness and a feeling of being more fully alive which involves all the three areas of human ability – thinking, feeling, and doing – coming together so that the spirit can live. Disabling any one part debilitates the whole, whereas acceptance enables a balanced involvement of each and is liberating.

Feelings are liberated by their acceptance. Unconscious attempts to control one set of feelings by picking and choosing those that will be allowed (these are good and those are not; these are judged acceptable and those are unconsciously considered undesirable; that one is so strong that it must be tightly held in), have the effect of splitting up the personality (Klein, 1952). Any superficial freedom 'to be' that might be gained by this splitting is limited by the 'no go' areas of secretly hidden parts that prevent openness and a real fullness of being.

Openness is restricted when people have an unconsciously pre-ferred, preconceived or given image of what is right and proper and good, an image that stands in the shadows of their unspoken past. Often, too, it is an idealized image; one which they cannot measure up to. A transient disillusion follows whenever it is let go, but disillusion, even transient disillusion, is a most unpleasant feeling. Disillusion: the loss of an illusion, in this case the illusion of the idealized self. The difficulty in taking this step is signalled by the many people who, instead, change their job, their house or their spouse.

However, turning once more to the patient/doctor scenario, the patient may experience the painful feeling of disillusion as he comes to see his doctor. Imagine a man who has always been fit and well. As a boy he took pride in his body. At school he derived great pleasure from playground competitions and thoroughly enjoyed a variety of team games. He became minutely aware of the bodily changes that signalled his move into adulthood and he made comparisons with the similar attributes of his school friends. As his body matured he derived satisfaction from the roundness of the muscles of his limbs and the play of sunlight in the fine hair that added a sheen to their surface. He would laughingly push out the muscles of his biceps with his thumbs so as to exaggerate them for team photos, but at the same time he proudly told himself that this was not necessary in his case. His body seemed never to let him down as he threw himself into all he did. With time this bodily self-image enabled him to have the self-assurance to talk with girls and eventually to ask one to go out with him. Step by step, on his physical body image all sorts of life experiences and perceptions began to build and take their place.

Over the succeeding years he had thought less about his body, and passingly believed this was because he was so busy in his work and with his new young family, but he once again recognized his own earlier feelings as he observed his children on the beach engaged in their various pursuits and mirrored by his son as he, in turn, grew up and matured.

But now he has come to see his doctor and is suddenly hearing that there is something seriously wrong with his body. He has not really, even passingly, thought about ageing with its loss of physical strength and failing abilities. His parents live far away and, in any case, are still fit and well, so that he has not had the experience of someone else's ageing thrust onto him through observing and hearing about it from people he holds dear. Suddenly, listening to his doctor, the pleasures and stature that his body had brought him and that have so warmed and satisfied him down the years seem to be about to slip away, and he senses that he can do nothing about it. His body, and with it his life, threaten to fall apart. Rather than face a growing realization of what the doctor has said, his mind races to find something to stop all this, to stop his having to face what, in its suddenness, seems to represent world-shattering losses. Then the doctor talks of a test to help him know what to do, and even though the doctor has previously said there is no cure, the man grabs hold of the idea of this test as if with both hands, not able at this point to consider the real and limited nature of what the doctor thinks might be gained by this option of 'help'. He dares not think of anything but cure, and as long as he does not face the limitations of what can be done for him, the doctor is likely to be thought of as being capable of reversing the disease processes. Suddenly the man becomes unreasonably dependent on his doctor, a dependency which is coupled with a god-like projection.

There is a dependency anyway when a doctor has knowledge and skills which a patient does not have for himself. There may be a further holding of a patient in an unnecessarily dependent position when a doctor does not share with a patient his knowledge of the options of treatment, nor educate him to enable him to make his own decisions. But, quite apart from these, there can be a projected expectation by the patient – as if a demand – that the doctor be all-powerful, and if the doctor succumbs to his own need to protect himself from the painful task of being present as a patient dismantles his defence, and if he does not firmly and gently help the patient to face reality and any resulting disillusion, projection's power takes hold. In these circumstances projection adds an extraordinary pressure and complexity to an already considerable and complex dependency.

To complete this picture it is necessary to look further than into the patient, and to what may be happening in the doctor. It can be an especially unbearable feeling for doctors to be impotent in the presence of another's psychological pain, and yet they must frequently face the inevitability of psychological distress and death, and their own disillusion at finding that their ability – both as a human being and as a doctor – is, in the final analysis, hopelessly limited. Rather than face this fully, a doctor may defend himself by attempting to deny reality and climb onto a pedestal labelled 'Excellent Carer'. He may make himself busy with excessively full care for the patient but, in the process, take over many of the responsibilities of the patient or the patient's family, even to the extent that his patient is left holding all the feelings of incompetence and powerlessness, while the doctor becomes vulnerable to the patient's projection that he be all-powerful. Ideally, a doctor talks so as to keep a patient as independent as he possibly can, but he still feels the demand and the desperate expectation that he be all-powerful and miraculously able to provide a cure. He is in medicine to help, so that this projection will often fall on fertile ground. When it does, it is a process in which both patient and doctor are involved, but it is the doctor who has the professional responsibility to steer the patient into grasping the reality of the situation and, therefore, it is up to the doctor to recognize the feeling of having been taken

hostage by the patient's feelings, and to divest himself of the unhealthy extra baggage of the patient's defensive and powerful projection. His job is to do this with a persistent, kind gentleness,
ready to face any resulting anger. It is better for both if the doctor
can acknowledge and share his own sense of uselessness and his
difficulty in merely observing.

This must surely be the aim because, for instance, for both
patient and doctor the acceptance of their own feelings, with all
the consequent conflicts they induce, is nonetheless followed by
an increasing trust in oneself and a sense of personal solidarity
and depth. There is a resulting understanding of the patient's
inner world, a world that is as real to them as the doctor's inner
world is to him, and each of their inner worlds is seen as separate
from any outside reality and, if anything, more important. It gives
the individual permission 'to be'. There is a 'letting-go' of the
need to control which releases energy for other uses. Freed to use
feeling, and with this extra energy now spare, the whole person is
available to be creatively involved with reality. Both doctor and
patient are set free.

However, and by contrast, persistent projectors are restricted by
the narrowness of the horizons that their attitudes and assumptions
impose. When one particular feeling is inevitably or continuously
projected, it results in the loss of that feeling, a devaluing of that
person's experience, and curtailment of his life. There is a loss of
independence and less of the person left to meet people in full
relationships.

Similarly, those who identify with a projection and are used by
others as a depository for 'unwanted' projected feelings are not
free to be themselves. It is as if other people's feelings nestle in
like a young cuckoo, so that the recipient is taken hostage by
forces that are not his own. These foreign feelings capture and
confuse him, squeezing out his own relevant and vital emotions
and reducing his self-awareness. It will therefore be seen that, for
both projectors and their 'victims', projection and projective identification so restricts their lives that it is as if they become, in
part, like dummies: the one devoid of their own ousted feelings,
and the other jerked about uncomprehendingly by other people's
feelings. At the extremes, their loss of freedom to be themselves
can be heart-rending.

It is better by far if a doctor works to return patient projections, but he will then be more acutely aware of his feelings in
relation to the reality of his work. While this has its rewards it is
also a difficult path to take, and to dwell for a time on some of
these difficulties will help to clarify the picture. For instance,

feelings produce conflicts, and many people find it difficult to hold conflicting feelings. It is as if they believe they must somehow have everything tidy and pulling all the same way, as if they must not allow themselves any confusion or internal discord. But feelings inevitably conflict, and if these conflicts are not accepted and worked with, they can seem to have a substance of their own which produces a shadow effect, stretching down the length of life. These shadows are repeatedly renewed by new situations mirroring those of the past, so that each somewhat similar but new predicament will, of a sudden, reproduce the past feelings, and to such effect that people can experience it as a repeat experience of the old. If only they could now resolve the conflict at last, they would be free to move on; if they cannot, those conflicting feelings will keep returning to swamp and enervate until such time as they are accepted. The need is for freedom to make a new beginning (Balint, M., 1968). If the past can be accepted unabridged, and its conflicting feelings valued as one's own, the present and future can also be faced.

Holding one's own feelings also necessitates the difficult work of adjusting attitudes so that feelings can remain part of one's conscious self. It can require considerable daring to let go of 'certainty' and the concrete, fixed self so as to relax into a flexible state, open to self-questioning and to change. This may seem impossible for those who need the security and certainty that comes from being told what to do, or of telling themselves they know what 'should' be done, and seem to know what is 'right'. In their need to relieve their anxiety, they attempt to find a place of safety by holding onto the skirt of another's authority, or by maintaining it in themselves.

Similarly, beliefs and attitudes can make it difficult for some to own their feelings. For example, some people believe it is self-centred for individuals to look to what they want. The judgemental overtone and projection involved in the words 'self-centred' whips both them and those around them into not spending enough time on themselves. Yet it is only if people work to be true to themselves that they can be whole and effective people, and their families, friends and acquaintances be supported to make that same journey. One person's freedom helps win it for another: patients are themselves empowered and enabled by the doctor reaching out for self.

Then there are other people who have difficulty because of the opposite belief: that life is a search for personal joy and pleasure. Often they hold onto this belief as if it were a 'right'. But an alternative belief to both these last two attitudinal stands is that life is full of interest and intriguing discovery, and is full of problem solving and involvement. Certainly life is a richly interesting experience that can more than occupy an entire life if only people will tuck into it and let themselves be involved. Sir Richard Attenborough's film, 'Shadowlands' (1994), portrays C.S. Lewis giving this an added dimension when he says that love is involvement.

There are commonly-held attitudes which also produce difficulties. Too often, tears are seen as a weakness rather than as merely an outward sign of a feeling that is a part of the self. Or a developmental 'breakthrough' to feelings is feared and regarded as threatening a 'breakdown'. Doctors can encourage people to grasp this freedom to feel, by themselves sharing in the process and neither colluding in making those with difficult feelings into scapegoats, nor turning to antidepressants to control them. There is a challenge for those around the patient to themselves be free, to move beyond thinking and action, and to include feelings. Doctors in particular will be helped and empowered in their work by being at home with their own full range of emotions. They will then find themselves appropriately referring patients more often to those trained to support and nurture this change.

One particular difficulty when holding one's own feelings occurs when faced with the grasping, spoiling nature of envy. Envy, greed and desire are frequently triggered by observing another person's freedom to be aware of their feelings and to be themselves. Uninhibited envy, jealousy or greed can produce claustrophobic, punishing imprisonment for the recipient, and people's malicious behaviour is often incomprehensible until this is understood (Fairbairn, 1952).

But there is an extra dimension to these difficulties for doctors. It has already been observed that the relationship between doctor and patient is one where projections onto the doctor are especially common, and his work with one patient after another often results in his being used in this way repeatedly. As a result he can be so overloaded with these recurrent experiences that his own defences are overpowered, and he may be thrown back in time to the feeling world of infancy, a time when he was enmeshed in a relationship of projection and projective identification. As an adult, however he finds this re-enactment, with its loss of identity, deeply disturbing. At the same time doctors who have been motivated to take up medical work because of a wish to relieve other people's pain and distress, and who hold a belief that they must be empathic with patients and experience the patient's feelings if they are to understand them, may experience these situations as if they are themselves taken hostage by their work.

Must doctors then refrain from seeking to ease the patient's burden by carrying some of it themselves? The answer here must surely be in knowing the feelings but being free to avoid taking them on oneself and, equally importantly, refraining from attempting to protect the patient. If, however, the doctor can recognize feelings and call them by their names, he can be reminded of instances when he has experienced them in his own life and recall something of what the patient is experiencing. This is quite different from taking on the patient's situation as if it were the doctor's own, to a point that he himself experiences the distress (or whatever the feeling is) of the patient's situation. He would then carry the patient's projected feeling as well as his own, so leaving him doubly loaded on the patient's behalf. These processes produce an unnecessary overload and one that it is essential for the patient to carry for himself if he is to be a full, independent and effective person. Protecting people from their own feelings is as unhelpful as protecting them from the realities of life and death, and simultaneously produces a burden that the doctor must learn to lay down if he is to be free to be himself.

These are some of the difficulties and attitudes that individuals may experience and which frustrate their sense of freedom. For those locked into circumstances such as these, an ability to adjust and relate more truly and intimately to others will, no doubt, slowly develop throughout life, but it will often come more quickly and fully through the experience of, as it were, being held safely while sorting through the present and the past in personal psychoanalysis or psychotherapy. I am clear that freedom to be creative with patients in family practice can be attained and that it is remarkably exhilarating, but it may well be that this state cannot be expected until the personal sort-out time of mid-life has largely taken place. Those who do refine their attitudes and abilities around this time may find that their newly released energies recompense them to some extent for the steady decline in their youthful energies, but in no way does it deal with the remaining problem of the excessive number of people who require such personal and demanding work. Too many patients demanding their doctor's attention for their human distress has a heavily debilitating result. For doctors the tiredness of excess workload too frequently, and often continuously, intervenes.

I would like to return to Brian Keenan's book, as his experience of being taken hostage has particularly spoken to me, and the extreme conditions of his experience brought him great clarity about the processes of projection. He gives a clear example and a memorable description of projection which I wish to end with. In his imprisonment, all nicety and superficiality were stripped away, leaving only the central core for his keen analysis. With great honesty and humanity he searches for meaning in his relationships with his jailers. Later in his captivity, and while still with John McCarthy, they were chained up in a barn-like building and separated from their guards by only a rough curtain so that they could observe their captors more closely. The book tells of his hard-won but increasing understanding of them.

He began to see that the guards produced fear in their captives to rid themselves of their own fear. Their brutal attacks on their prisoners were an unconscious attempt to grasp a sense of power and manhood for themselves, and had the effect of projecting and ridding themselves of their own feelings of weakness, vulnerability and despair. The hostages began to perceive their torturers' inner powerlessness and need for victims. It was then as if, by daring to fully feel the experience of being humiliated, dispossessed, powerless, vulnerable and deprived of rational thought to the point where they sometimes feared they were moving into madness, they could understand where these feelings really came from; could see them as belonging to their captors, and so come out the other side of these long drawn-out and horrendous experiences self-possessed and free of their guards' projections. With this understanding, they felt the torturers' own fear in the blows dealt to their bodies, and rediscovered their own power. Now they could resist by maintaining themselves internally, holding the boundaries of their personalities and shrugging off the guards' projections. They could joke and laugh at their torturers' vulnerability while still experiencing their own physical pain. Imprisoned, and in this most degrading and powerless of situations, these two men found an internal freedom.

> Even in those most deprived conditions we found within ourselves and within our shared discussions a more valuable and richer world than we had conceived of before. We were beginning to learn our freedom, the way Rousseau spoke of it. Captivity had re-created freedom for us. Not a freedom outside us to be hungered after, but another kind of freedom which we found to our surprise and relish within ourselves. (Keenan, 1992)

Even in the most dramatically distressing and exhausting human situation, personal freedom is fundamental, enriching – and achievable. For the doctor and the patient the issues may at first appear to be totally different to those of hostages and are cer-

166

tainly less dramatic, but for the doctor to do his job – and for both patient and doctor to live more satisfying and full lives – they, too, must join in and strive to find, and own, their feelings, leaving others to hold theirs, so that each can gain the freedom to be their full selves and, as Søren Kierkegaard puts it, 'be that self which one truly is' (1941).

APPENDIX 1

A Brief Autobiography

Many examples of personal and clinical practice have been outlined in this book and, because the nature of the doctor's work is so often discovered through his feelings, a self-knowledge in the professional worker is essential. That being so, it seems to me that the reader may find it important for his own awareness as he reads to know something of the background of the author. Here, then, is a brief outline to aid recognition of the attitudes and assumptions that may lie hidden in these pages.

I was born in 1936 in Ceylon (now Sri Lanka) to parents who had met there as missionaries. I was the third child, with an older sister and brother. The family returned to England when I was aged three, and we were home on leave when World War II began and when women and children were suddenly not allowed to travel. My father returned to Sri Lanka on his own, while my mother and we three children began a succession of moves between rented homes. Whenever a landlord's friends were bombed out of their home we would have to get out of his house to make it available for them. Consequently, there was a constant change of home, school and friends.

In 1947 my mother and I went back to Sri Lanka while my sister and brother stayed at boarding schools in England. I stayed there for two years, attending a boarding school in the hills. In 1949 we returned to England and I joined my brother at Kingswood, a Methodist boarding school in Bath.

I was clear I wanted to work with people, and chose medicine largely because of seeds sown by my mother. Both my parents now lived in England, moving every four years from church to church, as was then the norm in Methodism. In retrospect I must have been struggling throughout my early life to make sense of my repeatedly uprooted existence, as if it were a detective story or a puzzle, to find some framework that would give meaning to my reality.

After school I went to St George's Hospital Medical School at Hyde Park Corner, London, with the intention, after qualifying, of going as a missionary to a developing country. I met Ann at university, fell in love with her and we were married just as she began teaching and while I was still a student. I did my first hospital jobs at Warwick Hospital because of the rare married accommodation available there, and for two years I did a variety of jobs, all with an eye to working abroad.

In 1965, when we had two sons and a third child on the way, we set off to Eastern Nigeria and I worked at Ituk Mbang in a Methodist, two doctor, 200-bed bush hospital. The other doctor and I turned our hand to whatever was needed and whatever was of interest to us – as family doctor, hospital doctor, nurse's lecturer, pharmacist, architectural planner, building supervisor and business manager. There was a great deal to understand in what was going on around us, in a country that was building up towards the bitter, openly hostile phase of the Biafran war. We were involved in a lot of problem-solving to integrate modern medicine into the society in which we found ourselves.

My family and I returned to England in 1967, in part because I had now grown through my inner need to work abroad, and in part because it was clear our eldest son, John, now nearly six, was not responding to teaching, and there was no formal schooling available other than at a distant boarding school. It seemed to me that English general practice would allow the family to settle most quickly, and I chose a rural dispensing two man practice. I found the work limitless in quantity and it was lonely work, but at the same time it caught my imagination. Contact with other doctors was limited, and what there was seemed to be on a superficial level with no one admitting any difficulties. In the early 1970s I found a five-day course, organized in a small group format, where people could and did share their problems in their work, rather than maintain a front that allowed no difficulties and portrayed total control. My work now really opened up and I was excited by it.

There were no discussion groups running in my area where doctors could share their work experiences, so I started one. I also became involved with the general practitioner training scheme and the training case discussions. A general practitioner friend and I wanted to experience these as group members, and so we went weekly for two years to case discussion groups at the Tavistock Centre for Human Relations, North London (Gosling *et al.*, 1967). I now had confidence in the model and how these groups could function.

I am sure it is significant that during this time my wife and I discovered that not only our eldest son but all four of our boys had specific learning difficulties in the form of dyslexia. As my wife heard a description of the effects of dyslexia, she was saying to herself: 'That's John, that's just how he is.' At the same diagnostic interview, I found myself saying: 'But that's me, that's exactly how I am'. I now had a key to understanding my many failures in written exams. My sons and I were all formally tested and the condition confirmed. Here, I later realized, was another source of disconnected feelings, and a resulting need to find a linking structure for my experience. This discovery marked the beginning of a shift from a rather isolated struggle to function better into a wider understanding that everyone is joined in the struggle of life's endeavours, with each having their own particular brand of difficulty. I was not alone.

In 1983 I took a year's sabbatical. I had written to selected medical schools about my group work experience, and McMaster Medical School in Hamilton, Ontario took the bait.

This medical school was set up to explore the use of educational methods tailored for adults and described by Barrows and Tamblyn (1980). They did not aim to instruct the student, but rather to produce a climate for individual inquiry so that people discover for themselves. They seek to allow training to be self-motivated, and to enable the pleasure that self-discovery produces. Medical education at McMaster is not by lecture, nor by cramming what others have chosen should be inculcated, but by problem-solving experiences, usually in small groups and backed up by a large library of original research papers for the student to delve into, as and wherever his interest takes him.

I felt McMaster to be an ideal place to develop my teaching methods and, indeed, for my own development. For half my time I taught on a one-to-one basis or in small groups, and for the rest of my time had access to the various training courses run in small groups by the university. I studied the theory of education and involved myself in many different teaching situations to explore educational methods. I joined in with a rich mix of people, all applying the problem solving methods of adult education (Knowles, 1973) and also, of course, with the students and young doctors adjusting to their chosen work.

Returning to England, I wanted to extend this teaching experience and found myself drawn to psychotherapy work. I negotiated with my partner for the time necessary to enable me to train. I felt I could manage a day-release course, and selected my training accordingly at the Westminster Pastoral Foundation, London. Four years later I was awarded Diploma membership of the Institute of Psychotherapy and Counselling, validated by the Roehampton Institute. The course had involved me not only in that one day a week of course work, but also in my own case work with patients, the necessary personal study time and my own experience of analysis. There was, therefore, a lot of personal, theoretical and practical work and, as I live some ninety miles out of London, a great deal of travel. In retrospect, I can see that this not only increased my understanding of adult educational methods and of giving freedom to other people to explore but, through the training, gave me that experience for myself.

It should not have been a surprise to me that this training not only developed my counselling and therapy ability, but also opened up a whole parallel area of literature and thinking that has shaped much of medical practice, without doctors necessarily being aware of where it has come from. My family practice understanding and skills developed parallel to the course.

At the time of writing I work as a family practitioner, undertake formal weekly psychodynamic counselling of patients, am involved in counsellor training, am a Vocational Training Scheme general practice trainer and a course organizer for the day-release programme of the local Vocational Training Scheme course for doctors planning to enter general practice in the UK.

This, then, is the skeleton of my working life to date; the framework on which this book is built. It is from this, and through the many discussions with people who have shared themselves openly with me, that the ideas in this book have evolved. It is my approach and my way of looking at things today. Tomorrow – who knows?

APPENDIX 2

Useful Addresses

The following names and addresses may be useful. These organizations have been selected because of their relevance and/or established reputation for their standards in training. There are many more which can be obtained from the *Counselling and Psychotherapy Resources Year Directory*, obtainable from the British Association of Counselling.

Balint Society, Hon. Secretary, Dr D. Watts, Tolgate Health Centre, 220 Tolgate Road, London E6 4JS   Tel: 0171 474 5656

British Association for Counselling, 1 Regent Place, Rugby, CV21 2PJ Tel: 01788 550899

British Association of Psychotherapists, 37 Maplesbury Road, London NW2 4HJ   Tel: 0181 452 9823

Guild of Psychotherapists, 19b Thornton Hill, London SW19 4HU Tel: 0181 947 0730

Institute of Group Analysis, 1 Downs Road, Beckenham BR3 2JY Tel: 0171 431 2693

National Association for Patient Participation (NAPP)
11 Hardie Avenue, Moreton, Wirral, Merseyside L46 6BJ
Tel: 0151 677 9616

Relate Marriage Guidance
Herbert Grey College, Little Church Street, Rugby CV21 3AP
Tel: 01788 573241 (Also see your local telephone directory)

Society of Analytical Psychology, 1 Daleham Gardens, London NW3 5BY Tel: 0171 435 7696

Tavistock Clinic (Institute for Human Relations), 120 Belsize Lane, London NW3 5BA   Tel: 0171 435 7111

Tavistock Institute of Marital Studies, 120 Belsize Lane, London NW3 5BA   Tel: 0171 435 7111

Bibliography

The place of publication is London unless otherwise stated.

Allen, I. (1988) *Doctors and Their Careers*. Policy Studies Institute.
Balint, M. (1957) *The Doctor, his Patient and the Illness*. Pitman.
—— (1959) *Thrills and Regressions*. Hogarth.
—— (1968) *The Basic Fault*. Tavistock.
Balint, E. and Norrell, J.S. (1973) *Six Minutes for the Patient*. Tavistock.
Ballard, J.G. (1984) *Empire of the Sun*. Gollancz.
—— (1991) *The Kindness of Women*. HarperCollins.
Barrows, H.S. and Tamblyn, R.M. (1980) *Problem Based Learning. An Approach to Medical Education*. New York: Springer.
Belbin, R.M. (1981) *Management Teams. Why they Succeed and Fail*. Heinemann.
Berger, J. and Mohr, J. (1976) *A Fortunate Man*. Writers and Readers.
Berke, J.H. (1989) *The Tyranny of Malice*. Simon & Schuster.
Berne, E. (1968) *Games People Play*. Penguin.
Bion, W.R. (1959). 'Attacks on Linking', in *Second Thoughts* (1967). New York: Aaronson.
—— (1974) *Brazilian Lectures*, J. Saloman (ed.). Rio de Janeiro: Imago Editaria.
B.M.A. (1992) Report: *Stress and the Medical Profession*. B.M.A.
B.M.J. (1992) 'Sexual contact between doctors and patients' (editorial). *British Medical Journal* vol. 304. 13 June.
Bowlby, J. (1979) *The Making and Breaking of Affectional Bonds*. Tavistock.
du Boulay, S. (1984) *Cicely Saunders*. Hodder & Stoughton.
Bradbury, A. (1987) 'Anger as Therapy', in *Community Care* Haywoods Heath, 14 May 1987, no. 660.
Burnard, P. (1991) *Coping with Stress in the Helping Professions: A Practical Guide*. Chapman & Hall.
Cameron, N. and Rychlak, J.F. (1985) *Personality Development and Psychopathology. A Dynamic Approach*. Boston: Houghton Mifflin.
Campbell, J. (1988) *The Power of Myth*. New York: Doubleday.
Casement, P. (1985) *On Learning from the Patient*. Tavistock.
Cashdan, S. (1988) *Object Relations Therapy*. New York: Norton.
Erikson, E.H. (1977). *Childhood and Society*. Triad Paladin.
Fairbairn, W.R.D. (1952). *Psychoanalytic Studies of the Personality*. Routledge & Kegan Paul.
Field, J. (1952) *A Life of One's Own*. Penguin.
Fisher, F. (1992) Leader in *Medical Monitor*, 19 June 1992.

Fowles, J. (1969) *The French Lieutenant's Woman.* Jonathan Cape.

Freud, S. (1915). 'The Unconscious', in *On Metapsychology. The Theory of Psychoanalysis.* Pelican (1984).

Friday, N. (1981) *My Mother, My Self.* New York: Dell.

Frank, R. (1991) *Passion Within Reason.* New York: Norton.

Gosling, R. et al. (1967) *The Use of Small Groups in Training.* New York: Grune & Stratton.

Guggenbuhl-Craig, A. (1971) *Power in the Helping Professions.* Dallas: Spring.

Haslam, D. (ed.) (1994) *Not Another Guide to stress in General Practice!* Medical Action Communications Ltd.

Hess, H. (1972) *The Glass Bead Game.* Penguin.

Hodgkin, J. (1987) 'Who Helps the Helpers?' *New Society,* 1 May 1987, vol. 80, no. 1270.

Horney, K. (1946) *Our Inner Conflicts.* Routledge & Kegan Paul.

Jacoby, M. (1984) *The Analytic Encounter. Transference and Human Relationship.* Inner City.

Johnson, W.D.K. (1991) 'Predisposition to Emotional Distress and Psychiatric Illness Amongst Doctors: The role of unconscious and experiential factors', *British Journal of Medical Psychology* 64, 317–29.

Joseph, B. (1985). 'Transference: The Total Situation', *International Journal of Psycho-Analysis,* 66(4): 447–54.

Jung, C.G. (1964) *Man and his Symbols.* Aldus.

Keats, J. (1817) 'Letter to George and Thomas Keats 21 December 1817' in *The Letters of John Keats,* B.A. Forman, (ed.) (1941) Oxford University Press.

Keen, H. (1994) President, NHS Support Federation. Letter to *The Times,* 18 August 1994.

Keenan, B. (1992) *An Evil Cradling.* Hutchison.

Kegan, R. (1982) *The Evolving Self.* New York: Harvard University Press.

Kierkegaard, S. (1941) *Sickness Unto Death.* New York: Princeton University Press.

Klein, M. (1952) 'The Origins of Transference', in *Envy and Gratitude and other works* 1946–63. Hogarth.

Knowles, M. (1973) *The Adult Learner: A Neglected Species.* Gulf.

Knox, J.D.E. (1989) *On-Call.* Oxford Medical Publishers.

Lane, R.E. (1993) 'Why Riches Don't Always Buy Happiness' *The Guardian,* 9 August 1993.

Lao Tsu (1973) *Tao Te Ching. A New Translation,* G-F. Feng and J. English (eds), Wildwood House.

Lewis, C. Day (1977) *Poems of C Day Lewis (1925–72).* Chosen and Foreword by Ian Parsons. Jonathan Cape and the Hogarth Press.

Main, T. (1968) 'The Ailment', in *Cassel Hospital Book of Psychological Nursing.* Barnes.

Mainprice, J. (1974) *Marital Interaction and Some Illnesses in Childhood.* Tavistock Institute of Marital Studies.

Malan, D.H. (1979) *Individual Psychotherapy and the Science of Psychodynamics*. Butterworth.

Mattinson, J. (1975) *The Reflection Process in Casework Supervision*. Tavistock Institute of Human Relations.

—— (1979). 'The Deadly Equal Triangle', in *Change and Renewal in Psychodynamic Social Work*, Smith College School of Social Work. (1981).

McGregor, D. (1985) *The Human Side of Enterprise*. Penguin.

Menzies, I.E.P. (1970) *The Functioning of Social Systems as a Defence Against Anxiety*. Tavistock Institute.

Middleton, J. (1991) 'Helping the Practice Deal with Stress', *Pulse*, 23 November, vol. 51, no. 45.

Miller, A. (1985) *Thou Shalt Not Be Aware*. Pluto.

Neighbour, R. (1987) *The Inner Consultation*. Lancaster: MTP Press.

Ogden, T. (1982) *Projective Identification and Psychotherapeutic Technique*. New York: Aaronson.

Paul, N. (1975) *A Marital Puzzle*. New York: Norton.

Peters, T.J. and Waterman, R.H. (1984) *In Search of Excellence*. New York: Harper & Row.

Pincus, L. and Dare, C. (1978) *Secrets in the Family*. Faber & Faber.

Pritchard, P. (1993) *A practical guide to starting a patient participation group*. Royal College of General Practitioners.

Rayner, E. (1986) *Human Development*. Allen & Unwin.

Richardson, A.M. and Burke, R.J. (1991) 'Occupational Stress and Job Satisfaction among Canadian Physicians', *Work and Stress*, 5(4).

Rogers, C.R. (1961) *On Becoming A Person*. Boston: Houghton Mifflin.

Rutter, P. (1990) *Sex in the Forbidden Zone*. Mandala, Harper Collins.

Sanders, K. (1980) *A Matter of Interest*. Clunie Press.

—— (1991) *Nine Lives*. Clunie Press.

Searles, H.F. (1965) 'Problems of Psycho-Analytic Supervision' (1962b), in *Collected Papers on Schizophrenia and Related Subjects*. Hogarth.

Shaffer, J.B.P. and Galinsky, M.D. (1974) *Models of Group Therapy and Sensitivity Training*. New Jersey: Prentice-Hall.

Symington, N. (1986) 'The Analytical Act of Freedom as Agent of Theurapeutic Change', in *British School of Psycho-Analysis*, G. Kohon (ed.) Free Association Books.

—— (1986) *The Analytic Experience*. Free Association Books.

Watson, A.R. (1994) Chief Executive, British Association of Cancer United Patients. Letter to *The Times*, 18 August 1994.

Weatherill, R. (1991). 'The Psychological Realities of Modern Culture', *British Journal of Psychotherapy* 7(3) 268.

Wertheimer, A. (1986) *A Rotten Way to Die*. Society Tomorrow.

Wharton, E. (1920) *The Age of Innocence*. Penguin 1974.

Wilner, W. (1990) 'The Use of Primary Experiences in the Supervisory Process', in *Psychoanalytic Approaches to Supervision: Current Issues in psychoanalytic practice*, R.C. Lane (ed.), New York: Monographs of the Society for Analytic Training, no. 2.

Winnicott, D.W. (1975) 'The Manic Defence', in *Through Paediatrics to Psycho-Analysis*. Hogarth.

—— (1962) 'Providing for the Child in Health and Crisis', in *The Maturational Process and the Facilitating Environment*. Hogarth.

—— (1960) 'Ego Distortion in Terms of True and False Self', in *The Maturational Process and the Facilitating Environment*. Hogarth.

—— (1956) 'Primary Maternal Preoccupation', in *Through Paediatrics to Psycho-Analysis*, Hogarth.

—— (1941) 'The Observation of Infants in a Set Situation', in *Through Paediatrics to Psycho-Analysis*. Hogarth.

Woodhouse, D. and Pengelly, P. (1991) *Anxiety and the Dynamics of Collaboration*. Aberdeen: Aberdeen University Press.

Index

Indexed by Auriol Griffith-Jones